Health
and
Vitality Truths

Health and Vitality Truths
To Know and Tell

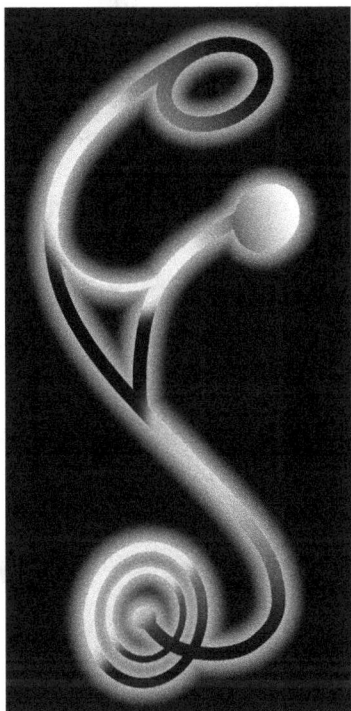

Luan Q. Pho, M.D.

Health and Vitality Truths
To Know and Tell

Luan Q. Pho, M.D., P.A.
1105 N. Central Expressway, Suite 260
Allen, TX 75013

Library of Congress Control Number: 2011913762

ISBN: 978-0-9837827-9-7

First Edition

Printed in the United States of America

Logo created by: William Owen

I dedicate this book to my father.

In memory of Cheryl,

and a special thanks to my patients,

my mother,

my wife Young,

and our three daughters –
Catherine, Emily, and Courtney.

Contents

Primum non nocere
Above all, do no harm!

Acknowledgements

I would like to thank those individuals who made this book possible. Thank you Diana for editing and for your help in getting this book on its way. A special thank you to Fred, Keith, Joe, and Aly for your time and valuable input. I also want to thank my patients who had motivated me to increase my knowledge in order to improve their health. Lastly, I want to thank my wife, who makes everything possible, and my three daughters who bring joy and happiness to our lives.

Warning and Disclaimer

The ideas, theories, concepts, opinions and clinical experiences expressed in this book are to be used for educational purposes only. It is intended to provide a different perspective on the subjects addressed in the publication. The nutritional information is designed to provide ways to achieve health and vitality. The reader should not adopt any of the suggestions in this book without first consulting with his or her medical, health or other competent professional. This book is not intended to replace any medical advice, provide diagnosis, prescribe or treat any disease, condition, illness or injury. It is sold with the complete understanding that the author and publisher are not offering or rendering medical, health, or any kind of personal professional services.

The author and publisher specifically disclaim any and all responsibility for liability, loss or risk, personal or otherwise, resulting as a consequence caused, alleged to have been caused by, directly or indirectly, from the use or application of any contents of this book.

When a man undertakes to create something, he establishes a new heaven, as it were, and from it the work that he desires to create flows into him...For such is the immensity of man that he is greater than heaven and earth.

– Philipus Aureolus Paracelsus

Preface

In writing this book, I am trying to make sense and understand the world we live in. As a doctor, I see patients daily who are suffering because their lifestyles have undermined their health. Although we have made huge strides in increasing the average lifespan, we are facing an epidemic of health problems related to obesity, our sedentary lifestyle and poor nutrition. *In this book, I will discuss what I call Micro/Macro Rx – the use of specific supplementation of nutrients and a healthful diet to help stave off many illnesses and chronic diseases.* I am writing to a lay audience, so my readers will be able to use the information to improve their health and vitality. Human illnesses and diseases and what we can do to prevent them will be discussed as well as exploring possible reasons behind a disease when the cause is currently unknown.

Trained in the field of Internal Medicine, I feel fortunate to have chosen a medical specialty that gives me a firm knowledge base to draw upon. I have a thirst for science and am most comfortable with medicine, my knowledge base and the profession I spend most of my waking hours involved in. My desire to learn accelerated after residency. During my "free" time, listening to audio books and podcasts broadened the scope of my knowledge. The educational podcasts were available as free downloads from the Internet. Listening to the podcasts and audio books was my gateway to a marvelous new world of information that would not have been possible otherwise.

I found the information to be new and informative. I was excited when a topic that I had recently listened to became relevant to my understanding of medicine. Listening, instead of reading, was my way to learn as much as possible. Information overload was never an issue. I wanted to absorb as much information as possible with the free time that I had.

In this book, I am connecting different bits of information in order to form a broader picture. This will enable us to make sense of the things that we do not currently understand since the connections are not readily apparent. I have tried to tie together the information from different fields of medicine so that it can logically explain the causes of illnesses and diseases that afflict so many of us.

A premise that I believe to be true is that with all the information currently available, we can solve many unknowns. The difficulties in this task will be gathering and understanding the many different and sometimes random pieces of information we come across -- i.e. information overload. There are times when what I say may actually raise more questions than those I have answered. But raising new questions from any discussion is beneficial.

I believe there are always possible answers to any question. Not finding an answer does not mean that one does not exist. The reason could be due to not asking the right question or not having all the information you need.

The answer to a question may come if you dedicate the time to think about the question and seek additional information in order for the answer to become apparent. When the answer does appear, it will appear as an "Aha!" moment. A quote that the psychologist Wayne Dyer stated during one of his inspirational talks, a quote that stuck with me is:

By believing passionately in that which does not exist,
we create it. That which is nonexistence has not been
sufficiently desired.

– Nikos Kazantzakis

This quote still resonates in my mind and is one of the driving forces behind my attempts to make sense of the world.

The materials contained in this book are based on what I have learned up to this point in time. The writing is a "work in progress." This means that the following information is not concrete since it reflects only my knowledge at the time of publication. The information may change in the future, especially if I am able to formulate new theories that are relevant to the topics I discuss in this book. My book seeks to incorporate insights from my work as a doctor and information from many different disciplines into a whole. By doing so, I hope to form a new hypothesis to explain many existing unknowns so readers can use the information to achieve optimal health.

I have done my best to document and cite the information used when it is not my own. In his book "Outliers: The Story of Success," Malcolm Gladwell states "People don't rise from nothing...They are invariably the beneficiaries of hidden advantage and extraordinary opportunities and cultural legacies that allow them to learn and work hard and make sense of the world in ways others cannot." This book reflects that concept. As with any advice or information you receive, you need to decide whether it is right for your particular situation. Critical analytical thinking is a difficult task due to the vast amount of information one receives daily. However, I sincerely want you to

think for yourself. Do not accept any information –
including mine -- as the "gospel truth." Ask yourself
where or how the person got the information he or she
is telling you. Try to seek and follow the information
trail for yourself. Once you do, what you might
discover could be very enlightening.

There is a lot of misinformation out there even
from so-called experts. I will ask that you read this
book with the same scrutiny I would when considering
any information given to me. For disclosure and
objectivity, the information discussed is my own, based
on my clinical experiences treating patients. My
theories are simply that – theories – and have not been
"proven" in clinical trials. *Any medical information
discussed may not be appropriate for you, and
you should always first consult with your own
physician*. As is often the case, professional or expert
opinions will vary since there are differing opinions on
any given topic.

The physician is only the servant of nature, not her master. Therefore, it behooves medicine to follow the will of nature.

– Philipus Aureolus Paracelsus

The Discovery

April 14, 2008. This was my date with destiny. It was the day my father passed away. On that day, I could no longer help him stave off the complications of Parkinson's disease. What I know now about health and vitality, I learned too late to help him. His time ran out before I knew what I needed to prevent the progression of his disease and untimely death. Looking back, I am filled with regret and longing. I wish I had had more time. I could have made a difference if only I had had more time. My father's death marked the beginning of my quest to find the answers that would improve the health of my family and patients. Less than two months later, I decided to start writing this book.

I remember April 14, 2008, as a warm pleasant spring day. I was attending a wound care course in the Woodlands, a suburb outside Houston, Texas. As an internist, I was interested in wound care because my father had pressure ulcers, a condition common in bedridden individuals. Pressure ulcers are caused by the constant pressure exerted upon the surface of the skin, usually at the bony surface of individuals who lack the capacity to relieve the pressure by movement. The pressure causes the integrity of the skin to give way and break down as an open sore. The main risk factor that predisposes individuals to suffer from pressure wounds is immobility.

In my specialty in wound care, I see and treat all different types of wounds. The patients I see in wound care, for the most part, are those whose wounds are not healing at all. The duration of these wounds can vary from acute to chronic. Most individuals with an open wound will heal without any problems. This is how most wounds work -- they are supposed to heal without any special attention except the usual care of keeping the wound clean and covering it with a bandage. However, among the patients I see in the wound care clinic, there is something that did not work right or else their wounds would have healed. This is where the mystery as to why a wound is not healing begins.

My job is to identify the cause or causes for a wound not to heal and fix it. If I can identify that reason, I can figure out the right treatment: My patients' wounds will then heal. The something that "did not work right," I soon discovered, is due in large part to the insidious lack of proper nutrition. Malnutrition often plays a significant role as to why a wound is not healing. Practicing wound care has enabled me to use my knowledge of nutrition to help heal wounds. Clinically, nutrition, when used in wound care and other aspects of life, has proven to be vital for health. *From my work in wound care and with other diseases, I now believe the single most important risk factor for illness and disease is malnutrition.*

Being alive is not the same as being nutritional healthy. This point should not come as a surprise to anyone, but I want to take it a step further: I believe individuals who lack the ability to heal their wounds almost invariably got that way due to some nutritional deficiencies. Nutritional disorders are divided mainly into two types: hypoalimentation (malnutrition or the lack of certain vitamins, minerals or macronutrients) or hyperalimentation (disorders such as obesity, caused by excessive macronutrient – eg. carbohydrates, proteins, and fats/lipids - consumption, rather than excessive intake of micronutrients – eg. vitamins and minerals).

Nutritional disorders involving protein intake include kwashiorkor (a form of malnutrition stemming from a lack of protein in the diet and often marked by a grossly swollen belly), marasmus (extreme emaciation and malnutrition in children), and catabolysis (the breakdown of fat and muscle tissue in order to stay alive), with each one representing an increase in the degree of severity.

Looking at the definition of catabolysis, one finds an interesting description. Catabolysis is a biological process in which the body breaks down fat and muscle tissue in order to stay alive. Catabolysis or catabolism is a destructive type of metabolism. It takes place when you are not supplying your body with the needed source of nourishment from proteins, carbohydrates, or fats, and it is the most severe type of malnutrition. It is especially interesting since the process of catabolism is similar to the autophagy process of cell death (the cell digests itself). The loss of muscle, subcutaneous tissue and fat sounds a lot like the etiology (cause or origin) behind the saran-wrap, paper-thin skin of elderly individuals who suffer skin tears.

For me, understanding the potential consequences of the nutritional disorders of malnutrition was as if someone had just turned on a light switch in my head where before there was only darkness and confusion. I may have heard such information years ago, possibly in biology class in college or in medical school, but I had failed to recognize its significance.

The general premise for the best possible health is that if you supply your body with all the micronutrients and macronutrients at their optimal amount daily, your body will use these nutrients efficiently and you will be healthy. This concept, in the simplest terms, is of supply meeting demands. The exact amount for most of the micronutrients and macronutrients needed daily is unknown or undetermined, because we are still thinking about nutrition in terms of food groups and serving sizes. Optimal nutrition is not about whether one is eating a low fat versus a low carbohydrate diet pattern. Optimal nutrition is about obtaining the needed amount of micronutrients and macronutrients that your body requires for you to achieve optimal health. Balance and moderation is the key. But how often is this achieved?

As I see it, every day you do one of two things: build health or produce disease in yourself.

– Adelle Davis

Truth #1

You Are What You Eat

You are what you eat. Yes, this is true. Believe me, when I tell you that this simple saying is the answer to the *secret to health and vitality.* The power hidden within these words is the Holy Grail, if you will, of health and vigor.

I have just told you the secret to optimal health in the beginning chapter of this book. Why have I chosen to do this? I could have kept it hidden until much later. But my goal is to give you the answers to as many questions about health and vitality as I can – and as quickly as possible.

The fact is that this well-known saying is too popular to be a secret. You might ask, "How can something so obvious be truly the secret to health and vitality?" The reason is that most of you know a lot more about the true answers to your health problems than you really want to admit. You might know what it takes to be healthy, but knowing the information and actually using it are two different things. I want to convince you to make the changes needed to improve your health and vitality. How successful I am in doing so depends on your appetite and desire to improve your health and vitality.

The work that lies ahead for me is to help you understand why the foods that you are eating daily will determine your health today and in the future. Most of us do not know where our food comes from except that we get it mostly from grocery stores. Once we buy it, we simply eat it, mainly for taste and without even considering how the food even got to us. The staggering variety, abundance, and convenience of foods available for our choosing have taken away the essential concept of why we eat. We went from eating for survival to focusing only on how the food tastes. The desire for inexpensive and good tasting food is a by-product of our current modern civilization. The reason you and I eat daily is so that we may stay alive. I say, "eat" but in reality, it is both eating and drinking water. For the sake of simplicity, from now on when I say, "eat," I am also implying "drink" (water). Eat and you will stay alive is a simple concept. It is so simple that I believe any reasonable individual would agree. However, for those few doubters known as breatharians, I can say with certainty that if you stop eating you will surely perish.

Now let's examine exactly what you are eating to stay alive. The majority of our foods are prepackaged and processed or have lost most of their nutritional value. They now have many extra ingredients and chemicals. Therefore, food choices are based upon availability, convenience, and cost (not necessarily in this exact order).

Your body receives the calories and nutrients from the foods you eat so you can function properly. But in order to be healthy, those calories must also have all the needed essential nutrients so that your body can use them to function at its best. This critical point cannot be stressed enough. In addition, we must consume enough of those essential nutrients in the proper daily amounts. Eating any one food or combination of foods does not guarantee that all the nutrients needed are available and consumed in adequate amounts for true health. *The lack of adequate amounts of any essential nutrients within the foods you consume will have significant implications for your health over the course of your life.*

You've probably heard the saying *"You are what you eat"* over and over from your parents, and maybe too frequently for your liking. Nevertheless, did you ever really understand it? It is ironic that such a simple statement holds the key to either health and vitality or illness and disease. If you are able to supply your body with all the needed essential nutrients in the proper amounts all the time -- and if you exercise regularly -- you will almost certainly be healthy. If you do not have the time to care about what you are eating and just eat whatever tastes good, your health will surely deteriorate over time. I certainly did not understand this until after my father's death.

I never really gave much thought into what it really took us to be healthy and vital. Our life seems to flow in an orderly way, yet in a fashion that we ultimately have no control over. One is born, grows old, and then dies. From the time you are born to the time you die, you stay alive by consuming food. Even so, food's potential for enhancing health and healing is not appreciated. The best time to maximize your health and vitality is when you are young, but when you are young, you often take many things for granted -- especially your health. It takes the wisdom that comes from aging to realize that optimal health is neither a guarantee nor everlasting. I am amazed why it has taken us so long to realize that such simple wisdom can have such an impact on our health and vitality.

We have yet to comprehend the significance of the fact that what we eat daily will affect our short-term and long-term health. We have twin epidemics of obesity and Type 2 diabetes in the United States, and more people are living longer with chronic health conditions. If we knew that the foods we eat daily hold the answers to health or illness, these diseases might not occur. In the following pages, I will try to unlock the powers that lie within foods. I will show you how to harvest the power of nutrition.

You can achieve health and vigor by eating foods that have the nutrients that your body really needs. Instead of eating foods just to satisfy hunger pains and the palate, consuming nutritious foods should be your goal. Yet ask yourself if you are doing this. You can do this by eating foods that fulfill a purpose and by obtaining any remaining nutrients you need through supplements. Supplementation is a good way to replace essential nutrients not readily available in natural foods.

That said, your health goals are up to you. If you want to be healthy and live a life as disease-free as possible, then eat the right foods. If health is not your main priority and you continue to do what you like, let me know when you are ready. I can still help. Keep in mind, though, after years of an unhealthy lifestyle, it is more difficult and may be even impossible to achieve optimal health.

Not having the right goal in mind is the reason most of us do not pay much attention to what we eat. Just think about it. Anyone can improve his or her health, irrespective of age, but this requires some effort once you understand nutrition. Health, at any one moment, reflects the prior decisions you have made regarding the foods you choose to eat, even decades earlier. Recent studies have shown that how lean someone is in his late teen's influences whether he will develop heart disease 20 years later.

Medicine is not only a science; it is also an art. It does not consist of compounding pills and plasters; it deals with the very processes of life, which must be understood before they may be guided.

– Philipus Aureolus Paracelsus

A Personal Account: Reversing Type 2 Diabetes Through Vitamin D Therapy

In science, the scientific method is the approach you use to test any hypothesis or theory. In medicine, clinical trials are used to test a theory or hypothesis. Anyone can have a theory, but what will determine if that theory works is whether it is can be reproduced by others and the result is the same each time. The topics that I'll be discussing may be factual or simply theories that will need further investigation by others before they are accepted. However, clinically, my experiences with the results in treating patients with vitamin D deficiency and tyrosine are nothing short of what could be called a miracle.

I have clinical evidence, for example, that vitamin D deficiency is an overwhelming causative factor for diabetes. The first piece of evidence is in the increased prevalence of vitamin D deficiency among people with diabetes – an association, to be sure, but a strong one. I have found, in fact, that all my diabetic patients are vitamin D deficient. The increased prevalence of vitamin D deficiency in people with diabetes does not establish a direct cause and effect relationship, of course, unless treating the condition of vitamin D deficiency can change a diabetic's blood glucose control. But this, in fact, is what I have seen when I started treating vitamin D deficiency in my diabetic patients.

In these patients, I found that treating the vitamin D deficiency improved their glucose control. The evidence I have regarding vitamin D as the direct causative factor in diabetes versus an association are in confirmed diabetic patients who either are off diabetes medication or have had their diabetes reversed by treating their vitamin D deficiency.

A diagnosis of diabetes is made in a number of ways. One way is by having a fasting blood glucose greater than 126 mg/dl on two separate occasions. Another way is having a blood glucose hemoglobin A1C (HgA1c) greater than 6.5. An individual's HgA1c is a value that correlates with their average blood glucose level for approximately three months duration. The management of diabetes rests on lowering an individual's blood glucose to as a normal range as possible or for an HgA1c level of less than 6.5 or at least 7.

There are different ways to achieve better blood glucose control. The cornerstone of diabetes management is lifestyle changes. However, this method is usually unreliable since it is fraught with compliance issue. The pharmacologic method to control blood glucose is with either oral diabetic medication or insulin. Insulin is the medication of choice for diabetics with an uncontrolled HgA1c or whose absolute number is greater then eleven. The reason insulin is used in diabetic patients with HgA1c of eleven or greater is because it is unheard of to lower an individual HgA1c to a goal of less then 7 without insulin.

In situations when insulin is not used or refused, then oral hypoglycemic medications are an option. There are many different types of oral diabetic medications available, all effective in lowering blood glucose. The effectiveness of each medication will vary. As a whole, oral diabetic medications when used in combination are only effective in lowering a person's HgA1c to no more than two and possibly three HgA1c points. For example, an HgA1c of 10 might be lowered to 7 or 8 with a combination of oral diabetic medications.

To have an HgA1c drop of more than 5 points is not documented anywhere in the literature when using only oral diabetic medications. Well, guess what: I have two diabetic patients whose HgA1c was lowered more than six points, (from twelve plus to less than six) with just one oral combination diabetic medication. An endocrinologist colleague presented one of my patients as a poster presentation at the American Society of Endocrinology annual meeting in Washington, DC in 2009! But how is this possible when I have just stated it was impossible for any oral diabetic medications, when used in combination, to bring down the HgA1C more than three points?

This is possible because in both of these diabetic patients, I recognized vitamin D deficiency and its potential role in causing diabetes. By actively correcting their vitamin D deficiency, I believed their insulin resistant state was reversed enough to reverse diabetes. If you still doubt that vitamin D deficiency actually causes diabetes, how about my third patient, a newly diagnosed diabetic? This third patient had an initial HgA1c of 11. He also had vitamin D deficiency. After hearing the experiences I had with vitamin D deficiency in patients with diabetes and discussing the treatment options, he elected not to take any diabetic medication but try lifestyle changes and have his vitamin D treated. In addition, he planned to monitor his finger stick blood sugar and follow up if any problems arose. After eight months, his latest blood testing for HgA1c had, amazingly, normalized from 11 to 5.5 without any diabetic medication. Again, how is this possible? This is possible because over an eight-month period his vitamin D deficiency was treated.

This patient did not take any diabetic medications. By just being on a low carbohydrate/increased protein diet and having his vitamin D deficiency treated, his HgA1c and blood sugar normalized. Had he only followed a course of lifestyle changes without having his vitamin D deficiency treated, I doubt that his blood sugar would have normalized. I believe that evolutionarily and by design, active 1-25-OH vitamin D plays a unique role in gene regulation that specifically controls glucose metabolism. With vitamin D deficiency, active 1-25-OH vitamin D role in glucose metabolism is hindered and presents as "insulin resistance."

The approach that I have taken in trying to make sense of the world of medicine is from a holistic approach. Merriam-Webster online dictionary defines holistic as: relating to or concerned with wholes or with the complete systems rather than with the analysis of, treatment of, or dissection into parts; holistic medicine attempts to treat both the mind and the body. A holistic or preventive approach is truly the approach that gives answers to health and vitality. Truly thinking holistically or preventively will put any personal, financial or political bias out of the equation. Having a personal, financial or political agenda often clouds one's judgments and ability to see the fact behind truths.

I believe that the science of medicine is a reductionist view. Medicine looks for answers to the causes of human illnesses and diseases from a reductionist view and not from a holistic view. This is evident by the many different medical specialties existing today. How can this type of reductionist viewpoint provide answers to human illnesses or diseases that require a broader view? Often, illnesses and diseases are managed symptomatically, since their origins are unknown. Illnesses and diseases can occur locally or systemically, but in order to understand their causes, you need to think globally. I believe that the best type of medicine is one that applies a holistic approach from individuals who have the knowledge of a reductionist.

With the vast amount of medical knowledge that exists, no one can know it all. Looking holistically at the world of medicine, I hope to broaden the scope of knowledge and give more answers than those that are known at this time.

The art of healing comes from nature, not from the physician. Therefore, the physician must start from nature, with an open mind.

– Philipus Aureolus Paracelsus

Truth #2

Prevention: Why is it Important to Your Health?

The desire to stay healthy and to age well is the reason I am seeking to find the keys to healthy and vitality. As a son of a father who died from Parkinson's disease, I have witnessed the many difficulties that accompany a chronic illness. I have experienced the powerlessness and despair of watching my father and some of my patients die. During the years that my father had Parkinson's disease, I was not able to slow down the progression of his disease. I watched helplessly as he declined from one complication after another.

It was during the final days of witnessing my father's suffering that I made a commitment to discover the cause or causes for Parkinson's disease. At the very least, I felt I could try. If I ended up not finding the cause for Parkinson's disease, then I would try to seek ways to slow down its progression. Confronted with his misery and eventual death, my own mortality and that of other loved ones became real. I wondered if I too would develop Parkinson's disease, and if so, could I stop it? Better still, could I prevent it from happening to me? Would I be as helpless in facing the same disease and suffering that I witnessed in my father?

The goals of trying to discover the cause or causes for Parkinson's disease sounded like an insurmountable task. Yet it is a goal I had confidence that I could achieve. I felt the answers to what causes Parkinson's disease were within reach, because there is always a cause and an effect to everything in this world. Parkinson's disease is the effect. What I had to discover was the cause. I realized that others have tried and are still trying to achieve this same goal. So why did I feel that I could even attempt to find an answer that currently does not exist? The reason is that when confronted with the death of a loved one, one's own mortality comes into question.

If I wanted to slow down the devastation of Parkinson's disease, I felt that the answer would not be found by trying to identify the cause directly. One way to approach finding the cause for Parkinson's disease, or any disease, is to discover how to live without a chronic illness. *Illness and disease are the opposite of health and vitality*. Therefore, the way to discover the causes for illness and disease is to find the answers to health and vitality.

The advantage to this approach is unlimited. Unlocking the keys to good health would not only help me but also my family and my patients. After the death of my father, the thought that crossed my mind was that another family member, perhaps even me or my daughters, might suffer from Parkinson's. It was a fate I deeply wanted to avoid. This fear strengthened my desire to fulfill the promise that I made to my father: to find the cause of Parkinson's disease.

To find the cause for a dreaded illness: what could be a better goal? In working on it, I could help my patients, my family and myself. This was truly a win-win situation for everyone. My plan was simple and straightforward. Apply the knowledge that I already had to the information that I would need to learn. From this, I would then have to come up with the answer to the question as to how an individual can achieve optimal health and vitality. I started my quest by concentrating on research about Parkinson's disease, especially findings not considered as the norm. By making connections between what I learned and what I already knew, the answer, I hoped, would then become apparent.

I devoted my time to thinking about the big picture regarding health and disease. For me, the challenge was to understand not only health but also events that lead to that state. As an internist, I am trained to diagnose illnesses and diseases through signs and symptoms. For instance, patients typically come in (or in doctor speak, "present") with a chief complaint, which is a sign or symptom of an illness or disease. From these signs and symptoms, I have to figure out the likely diagnoses that best explain them. Signs and symptoms that match to a medical descriptive word equal diagnosis. Once a diagnosis is determined, I have the option to prescribe or not prescribe a medication. Prescription medications are a modern day medical miracle, since they will usually ease or relieve symptoms.

The benefits of prescription medications are undeniable. Medication is something we all like to have available when we are sick. However, using prescription medications may not treat the underlining reason for your illness. The real answers for the root causes of most diseases are the same as the keys to good health. To treat the symptoms of an illness is not treating its root cause, but only its signs. This approach is similar to putting a bandage on a cut. The bandage will stop the bleeding but does nothing to prevent the cut from happening again.

Let's take a look at how medicine defines preventive health. The U.S. Preventive Services Task Forces' Guide to Clinical Preventive Services defines primary prevention as measures provided to individuals to prevent the onset of a targeted condition. Primary preventions   -- which include immunizations and health education -- are meant to help you avoid a given illness or disease. Primary prevention is successful in helping avoid or alleviate the suffering, cost and burden associated with a disease; indeed, it is the most cost-effective form of healthcare.

Activities that identify and treat at-risk individuals who have no symptoms in order to prevent an illness or disease from occurring are called secondary preventions. This form of prevention targets those who already have developed preclinical disease or risk factors yet whose conditions are not clinically apparent. These activities focus on early detection of the asymptomatic disease that has significant risk for negative outcomes without treatment.

Secondary preventive measures work best when there is a significant latency period for the disease screened. Examples include screenings such as tests for high cholesterol, high blood pressure, and breast cancer. With early detection, the natural history of the disease and its effects over time is altered to minimize suffering and maximize health.

Tertiary prevention involves the care for individuals who already have an established disease. Such prevention attempts to restore function, reduce the negative effects of the disease, and prevent disease-related complications. Once the disease is present, primary prevention activities are not attempted or not successful even when tried. Tertiary prevention, in fact, is a misnomer because it does not actually prevent disease.

The relationship of signs and symptoms and how they are related to other diagnoses are generally not considered when any one diagnosis is made. When a given diagnosis is made from a set of signs, symptoms, physical findings or blood tests, the scope of knowledge becomes narrower. My interest in health is not to treat the sign, symptom, or physical findings. My interest is to identify the root cause of the illnesses or disease states. This will enable me to better practice preventative medicine.

Preventing illnesses or diseases from occurring -- or primary prevention -- is a professional goal that I had when I started to practice medicine. Currently, nothing exists that I know of that is able to prevent the progression of Parkinson's disease. I want to find that what "does not exist." This will enable me to truly practice preventive medicine.

Preventive medicine is not one of the strengths of traditional allopathic medicine. I say this not as a criticism of the system of which I am a part, but as an observation of how I see medicine as it exist today. Allopathic doctors are trained to do exactly what they are doing -- that is, to diagnose and manage illnesses and diseases with diagnostic testing and prescription medications.

In terms of diagnosis, I believe that allopathic doctors are competent and are doing the job that they are trained to do. In the aspect of managing or preventing disease, I believe that the allopathic training that a doctor receives is failing them and their patients. Allopathic doctors are trained to diagnose signs, symptoms, and physical findings. Blood tests are also used to aid in the diagnoses. Prescription medications are then used to treat the illnesses. Allopathic doctors are not trained to identify the root cause of diseases. They are trained to treat a given illness or disease with prescription medications, but that will not lead to health and vitality.

The medical education that allopathic doctors lack is the diagnostic skill to identify and treat nutritional deficiency. The diagnostic skill that is missing is the ability to interpret illness not as an isolated entity but more holistically. The main part that is missing in the allopathic training is nutrition education. Nutrition education should be a key component of preventive medicine. Nutrition holds the answers to health and vitality.

The current medical system is at a crisis point due to the rising cost of healthcare, which has skyrocketed due to the cost of taking care of individuals with chronic medical diseases. During his presidential campaign, President Barack Obama stated, "This nation is facing a true epidemic of chronic disease. An increasing number of Americans are suffering and dying needlessly from diseases such as obesity, diabetes, heart disease, asthma and HIV/AIDS, all of which can be delayed in onset if not prevented entirely." I agree with this assessment. However, the treatment of a disease once it is symptomatic is not really treating the disease but just treating its symptoms. The ultimate goal is to practice primary prevention.

This is particularly important today, since the average human life span for a person living in the US is about 77.9 years. This data comes from the National Center for Health Statistics (NCHS). Life expectancy increased dramatically in the 20th century, especially in developed countries. In 1901, life expectancy at birth in the United States was 49 years. By the year 2000, it was 77 years, an increase of 57%. Similar gains are happening in other parts of the world. In 1950, life expectancy in China was only around 35 years. By year 2000, it had risen to around 71 years. In

India, life expectancy in 1950 was around 32 years; by 2000, it had risen to 64 years.

The increase in the number of years of life expectancy is due largely to the eradication and control of infectious diseases. In addition, technological advances have made treating illness possible in cases of conditions that would have killed us in the past. Instead of dying from infection, we now have antibiotics to treat those very infections that once would have proven fatal. However, this has not come without a price. Instead of dying at a younger age, we are now dying from diseases or processes that are slow and chronic in nature, such as heart disease, diabetes, and cancer. Currently, the two leading causes of human death are cardiovascular disease and cancer.

One obstacle to primary prevention of such diseases is the need to convince individuals without signs of illness that they should take active steps to improve their health. Trying to convince a person to take pro-active steps for health is like talking about personal responsibility, something we all think we possess more of than we actually do. Another obstacle in primary prevention is that you are trying in theory to prevent something that might or might not even happen.

In medicine, the etiologies of most illnesses or diseases are still unknown. When the cause for an illness or disease is not found, we label it as "iatrogenic," a medical term for an unknown cause. As we get older, when an illness or disease strikes, the cause of the condition is often blamed on age as often as iatrogenic is labeled as the cause when you are younger. The aging process is undeniable. How well you age is the real issue as to whether an illness or disease will arise at that age. For every disease thought to be simply due to age, I believe the real culprit is usually due to a lack of proper nutrition throughout one's life.

The future of medicine needs to head towards primary prevention if the goal is to reduce the burden of chronic diseases. Identifying root causes of diseases will help prevent those diseases from occurring and lead to improved health and vigor.

I tell my patients that I can treat their diseases by prescribing the appropriate prescription medications. These medications, in the short term, will get them better or reduce their symptoms. However, by just using traditional prescription medications, their underlying diseases will still persist and continue to progress over time. To reverse the "natural" progression of a disease is to look not at the disease but to identify factors that maintain your health, strength and energy.

In using a tree as an analogy, think about illnesses and diseases as its branches. Each branch of the tree will represent an illness and then disease. The trunk of the tree represents health and vitality. When you are able to move ever closer towards the trunk of the tree, you will have identified the core or root defect of a disease. Moving towards the trunk of the tree and towards the "root causes" is the goal for health and vitality.

Once a disease has entered the body, all parts which are healthy must fight it: not one alone, but all. Because a disease might mean their common death. Nature knows this; and Nature attacks the disease with whatever help she can muster.

– Philipus Aureolus Paracelsus

Truth #3

Nutrition: The True Fountain of Youth

The goal of nutrition education is to teach that health is achieved through moderation and a balanced diet. I agree and would stress that the concept of a balanced diet is the answer to health and vitality. However, a moderate and balanced diet is not what most of us are eating.

When one talks about a balanced diet, the important point to consider is, "What are you trying to balance?" Is it the actual foods eaten, or is it the macronutrients (carbohydrates, proteins, fats) found within the foods that are important? Optimal health should require a diet pattern not only balanced in the macronutrients consumed, but also of the quantity needed.

For years, nutritional education has focused on the food pyramid system as a starting point. The United States Department of Agriculture (USDA) governs the information within the food pyramid system, which is based on five main food groups. Although the increasingly unwieldy food pyramid has just been replaced with a new icon called MyPlate, which stresses eating smaller portions, avoiding sugary drinks, making sure half your plate consists of fruits and vegetables, and eating whole grains, I will focus on the food pyramid because it had been in use for decades and has arguably had the greatest impact on current dietary patterns.

The five different food groups that make up the food pyramid system are meats, dairy, fruits, vegetables and bread/cereal/rice/pasta. Currently, the prevailing nutritional advice is that you should eat 2 to 3 serving of meats, 2 to 3 serving of dairy, 3 to 4 serving of fruits, 3-5 serving of vegetables and 6-11 servings of either bread/cereal/rice/pasta daily.

The food pyramid system deals in food groups and not the micro and macronutrients found within the foods that it represents. It focuses on the physical form of foods when it really should be on the actual nutrients themselves, since they are the key to health. The physical forms of the foods eaten do not matter as much as the nutrients they represent.

So what is the answer to increased health and vigor? Eating more or fewer foods is not the answer. The key lies in knowing what to eat. You need to know how to obtain the essential micro and macronutrients and the amount needed daily. This is a very important point that the food pyramid system fails to consider. The reason for this is that current nutritional thinking pushes a philosophy of food groups and not the essential micro and macronutrients you need. When you are eating to get sufficient nutrients, you will not ask how many food servings to eat but the amount of the actual micro and macronutrients needed. The amount of nutrients you need, in turn, depends on your body weight. Using body weight as the determining factor in figuring the daily amount of nutrients needed is the first step to health.

Another issue with the food pyramid nutrition education is that most individuals believe it and yet cannot follow it. In order to overcome this, you have to recognize the deficiencies within the food pyramid system. For you to achieve optimal health, remember that the concept of a balanced diet as the way to health is sound.

If you read on, I will focus on the micro and macronutrients essential for health. You will then have the keys to optimal nutrition, which will equate to improved health and vitality.

Here's a brief summary of what you need to know:

When you eat, what your body does with foods is to use the digestive mechanisms in your stomach to break them down into these five basic nutrients: carbohydrates, proteins, lipids, vitamins, and minerals. These five nutrients make up the micronutrients and macronutrients essential for life. Your body does not view the foods you consume in terms of the five food groups or necessarily care if the recommended servings were consumed. What is important regarding nutrition is whether you have consumed enough of the five essential nutrients daily or not.

These five essential nutrients need to be available in adequate amounts for your body to function properly for the moment, the minute, the hour, and the day. The nutrients discussed are terms that all of us are familiar with. What may be new is the concept of thinking about nutrition in the terms of food nutrients and that our daily requirement is dependent upon our body weight and metabolic demand. By using these terms and thinking about nutrition in these terms, it is easier to identify what may be potentially missing or deficient from our everyday diet.

Think about nutrition in terms of carbohydrates, proteins, lipids, vitamins and minerals. Then ask yourself if you are getting enough of these nutrients daily for your body weight and for what your body needs. If you are unsure how much you should be getting, don't worry: I will explain that in detail in subsequent chapters. The other nutrient that is essential for life is water -- the sixth nutrient needed for life. However, most people know to drink 6 to 8 glasses of water daily, so we can just concentrate on food.

The macronutrients are made of carbohydrates, proteins, and fats/lipids (CPF). These macronutrients not only serve as an energy source but also play a critical role as building blocks for our cells. Each of the macronutrients will serve a diverse role in your overall health but I will try to over-simplify each macronutrient to what I believe is its main function. The main role of carbohydrates --specifically, glucose -- is as an energy source that our body uses to convert the stored energy into adenosine triphosphate (ATP), the actual energy currency of our body. Proteins, as a macronutrient, consist of twenty amino acids, which are the building blocks that our cells use to build enzymes and critical brain neurotransmitters. The main role of lipids is as an energy storage form for extra calories. Lipids are calorie dense, meaning they have more calories per gram, compared to proteins and carbohydrates.

When you consume excessive dietary calories, either as carbohydrates or as protein, your body will convert these extra calories into fats. Remember, you eat for two reasons. The first is to keep you alive. Foods functioning in this capacity are similar to the gasoline that powers a car's engine. Any of the macronutrients -- carbohydrates, proteins, or lipids -- can serve in this role. The second reason we eat is to supply our body not just with an energy source but also with the essential building blocks needed for proper health. Again, the macronutrients -- along with micronutrients --play an important role in this function.

Micronutrients are vitamins and minerals, including antioxidants. These important nutrients are needed for cellular metabolism to occur properly. Cellular metabolism encompasses the synthesis, repair and/or replacement of existing cells. During cellular metabolism, antioxidants help by acting as hydrogen donors. They also help your body deal with the waste created by cellular metabolism or cellular damage. You can think of antioxidants as the garbage truck that carries garbage and waste away from your home.

These explanations are a very over-simplified way of explaining micronutrients and macronutrients, and they don't include all of their functions. Nevertheless, the one thing that is true for both micronutrients and macronutrients is that our body requires each nutrient in a certain amount daily. *The lack of a micronutrients or macronutrients in the amount needed is the cause for illnesses and diseases.*

Consider the building blocks of nutrition to be micronutrients and macronutrients, instead of the food pyramid. What becomes apparent is that the potential for deficiencies in micro- and macronutrients is real. It is real due to what we are choosing to eat everyday.

The likelihood that deficiencies will occur depends on the amount of carbohydrates, proteins, lipids, vitamins, and minerals consumed versus what is actually needed. For example, we do not consume enough of certain fats, specifically the essential fatty acids known omega-3 fatty acids. With inadequate daily intake, deficiencies of any particular nutrients will likely worsen over time.

The macronutrient most likely consumed in over-abundance is carbohydrate. The macronutrient most likely consumed in an insufficient amount is protein. Deficiencies of micro or macronutrients cause ill health. Similarly, over abundant intake of a particular macronutrient can also undermine our health. The detrimental health effects from the over-consumption of carbohydrates are in part due to how our body has to adapt to this surplus.

A balanced diet that provides the optimal amount of essential micronutrients and macronutrients is effective in achieving health and vitality in a true "Fountain of Youth." I use the term "Fountain of Youth" not to imply that anyone can or should live forever. Nevertheless, optimal nutrition will enable you to be healthier and live longer then otherwise possible, and lowers the probability of you having any type of chronic illnesses or diseases. However, no single one nutrient or combination of nutrients is ever the answer to optimal health. The Fountain of Youth concept doesn't embrace a single pill or a magic portion that one can just take and expect to be healthy. It is the concept of fulfilling the body's daily requirement of the basic essential micronutrients and macronutrients needed.

In the following chapters, I will discuss each of these five nutrients -- carbohydrates, proteins, lipids, vitamins, and minerals -- in more detail. I'll then examine diseases connected to vitamin D and protein deficiency, and will finish by making an argument that you will need to supplement your diet if you want optimal nutrition.

Carbohydrates

It's likely that you eat too many carbohydrates since they are all around us. Carbohydrate foods are the by-products of a modern civilization that craves convenient, fast, and inexpensive good-tasting foods.

The current Acceptable Macronutrient Distribution Range (AMDR) for carbohydrates that you should eat daily is from 45% to 65% of your total daily caloric intake. In a 2000 calories daily diet, this is about 225 grams to 325 grams of carbohydrates a day. This recommendation, unlike that for proteins and fats, does not vary depending on your age.

Each gram of carbohydrate is able to provide four kcal of energy. Carbohydrates have the general molecular formula of CH_2O. This means that the basic molecular structure for all carbohydrates will have a carbon atom, two hydrogen atoms and an oxygen atom. The actual number of carbon, hydrogen, and oxygen atoms will vary depending on whether the carbohydrate is a simple sugar known as a monosaccharide versus a disaccharide, which are two sugars connected to one another. Examples of monosaccharide sugars are glucose, galactose, and fructose. When a monosaccharide is linked together to a monosaccharide, you then have a disaccharide such as sucrose, maltose and lactose. A polysaccharide is a chain of monosaccharide or disaccharides linked together.

Sucrose, also known as table sugar, is a glucose and fructose linked together. The major sugar in milk is lactose and is formed from glucose and galactose. Maltose has two glucose molecules bonded together and is the constituent of starch. Starch has multiple maltoses bonded together in a long chain to make up a polysaccharide. Foods that are polysaccharides are corn and potatoes. During starch digestion, glucose molecules are released and absorbed into your bloodstream. The speed at which starch is digested and glucose is absorbed into your bloodstream will vary depending on the source of foods eaten. The glucose from foods that are high in the glycemic index – a table that measures the effects of carbohydrates on blood sugar levels -- will be absorbed faster into your bloodstream and tend to cause higher insulin release when consumed.

Carbohydrate is an important macronutrient since your body uses glucose as its main fuel source to keep you metabolically alive. In fact, your brain uses glucose as the preferred source of energy. It is believed that your brain's requirement is about 120 grams of glucose a day, or about 24% of your daily total energy expenditure. The rest of the glucose consumption is then used to fuel your organs, muscles, and red blood cells. As such, glucose is an important nutrient needed for your survival.

The blood glucose level within your bloodstream is tightly regulated within a narrow range by two opposing regulatory hormones: insulin and glucagon. Insulin is released from the pancreas in response to your blood glucose level. The action of insulin is to lower the blood glucose level back toward the normal range. When the glucose level in your blood becomes too low, glucagon will be released. Glucagon's action is to raise the blood glucose back to normal once the glucose level goes below what is normal for the particular person. Glucagon also breaks down glycogen into glucose. Glycogen is a polysaccharide, a chain of glucose.

The propensity for insulin or glucagon's release and action are dependent on what your blood sugar levels are throughout the day. Since your blood glucose goes up after a meal, insulin is released to bring it back down towards the normal range. If your blood glucose is too low, because of exercise, skipped meals or for other reasons, then your body will release glucagon to release glycogen. Glycogen will raise your blood glucose level because glycogen is your body's stored glucose.

Glycogen, in fact, is your body's first line of defense against low blood glucose. For prolonged hypoglycemia or during periods of not eating, glycogen's role is to serve as a short-term back-up fuel source. Once glycogen levels become low, your body will then begin to break down proteins and lipids as the other source of fuel. The energy potential for a carbohydrate is the same as for a protein, with each providing about four kcal per gram of energy.

Cellulose is another type of carbohydrate, but unlike the carbohydrate that was just discussed, it is not digestible by humans. Cellulose is fiber and is found in grains, vegetables and the fruits we eat. Since we are not able to digest cellulose, it does not contribute any energy in the form of food calories. Cellulose, in the form of fiber-based foods, aids in digestive health. Fiber provides feelings of satiety by slowing the progression and emptying of foods from your digestive system.

A diet high in carbohydrates can have adverse effects on your body. One adverse effect is that you may not consume enough of other macronutrients such as proteins and lipids. *You should always have a diet that is reasonably balanced in terms of macronutrients.* Yet, a diet typical of the one found in the food pyramid is imbalanced toward carbohydrates. This imbalanced consumption of macronutrients is the root cause of illnesses and disease. A diet based on fruits and vegetables is really a carbohydrate diet, because when the fruits and vegetables are broken down into their micronutrients and macronutrients element, they are mainly composed of carbohydrates, fibers, vitamins and minerals.

Another adverse effect of a high carbohydrate diet is due to the response created by eating a meal that is high in sugar content. A high glucose meal will cause an increased release of insulin. In addition, since your body regulates glucose within a narrow range, any increase in blood glucose above a set range will cause a change in metabolism, resulting in your body storing glucose as fats.

Either the form or the amount of carbohydrates consumed will affect the rate of carbohydrate metabolism and its conversion to lipids. The insulin release associated with eating a high glycemic index carbohydrate is greater than that of a low glycemic index food ("fast" and "slow" describe how quickly the carbs break down in the body). The greater amount of glucose quickly digested and absorbed is the reason your body starts storing glucose as fats. Eating excessive carbohydrate calories can make you obese due to the effects of insulin action on glucose. All carbohydrates consumed are used immediately or are stored as reserve energy, first as glycogen and then as body fat. Therefore, a high carbohydrate diet, day in and day out, will lead to obesity if the total caloric intake is greater than what your body needs.

Proteins

The current recommended daily allowances (RDA) of protein intake that you should consume each day varies from 5%-35% of your total daily caloric intake. For children ages one to three years old, the recommended daily protein intake is 5%-25%. For children ages four to eighteen years old, the recommended daily protein intake increases to 10%-30%. The adults' recommended daily protein intake is 10% -35%.

Protein is one of the three macronutrients needed for your body to function properly. Proteins serve as a fuel source for your body, similar to that of carbohydrates and lipids. When you deplete your body's blood glucose by physical activity, your body will start breaking down other forms of stored glucose, such as glycogen. Once the body's glycogen storage is depleted, the next source of fuel used is the proteins and then lipids. Your body is able to convert proteins and lipids into glucose through a process call gluconeogenesis. From a fuel standpoint, the preferred fuel source is glucose, glycogen, proteins, and lastly fats.

Besides serving as an energy source, the amino acids found in proteins serve as key nutrients in functioning as the building blocks of your body. Amino acids also serve as precursors for key hormones, enzymes, receptors and neurotransmitters in your body. *In my opinion, unlike carbohydrates and lipids, proteins are the most important nutrient needed to maintain your health.* An over simplified explanation for the function of carbohydrates and lipids is that they mainly serve as an energy source to "run your body's engine." The role of proteins involved in your health is different in that it serves as your body's main building blocks.

Your body is composed of about 20% protein by body weight. Protein is the nutrient that forms all your structural tissues and organs. It can function as a fuel source in time of scarcity of carbohydrates or fats. Protein is the main nutrient that your body uses to maintain itself so that you will not break down today, tomorrow or in the distance future. It maintains your health the way a well-maintained car engine preserves the car's longevity.

Protein is made up of twenty different amino acids. Each gram of protein is able to provide four kcal per gram of energy. They are long chains of amino acid connected to one another by a peptide bond. Proteins are similar to a long sentence, with each word being an amino acid. A protein can be hundreds to thousands of "words" long.

Your body needs an adequate amount of proteins daily so that it has all the essential and non-essential amino acids needed for cell maintenance, cell repair, or cell replacement. When all the essential and non-essential amino acids are contained within a particular food consumed, then this food is considered a complete protein. Amino acids are released during food digestion by enzymes that break down the peptide bonds that hold the amino acids together. Amino acids are the building blocks of tissue proteins, which comprise approximately 20% of your body weight (about 13.5 kg in a 70 kg man). During the process of protein digestion, up to twenty amino acids are released.

The twenty amino acids that make up the protein within the foods we eat are either essential amino acids or non-essential amino acids, depending on whether we can synthesize it in our body. The essential or non-essential label of an amino acid does not have anything to do with whether your body needs it for survival or not. Your body needs all the twenty amino acids for survival and for proper health. In most cases, the nonessential amino acids are synthesized from the essential amino acids if you have consumed enough of the essential amino acids. If you have not consumed foods that have all the essential amino acids daily, you will eventually become deficient in not only those essential amino acids but also the nonessential amino acids. *Once the pattern of inadequate protein consumption becomes chronic – for either the essential amino acids or the quantity needed for one's body weight -- the potential ill effects from the lack of a particular amino acid needed for proper health will show up as illness or disease.*

The nine essential or "indispensable" amino acids are histidine, isoleucine, leucine, lysine, methionine, phenylalanine, threonine, L-tryptophan, and valine. Your body is unable to synthesize these amino acids, and thus the daily availability of these amino acids is dependent on your diet. When you eat foods that do not contain these essential amino acids or the amounts are inadequate, you will be deficient in the essential amino acids for your daily metabolic needs. When this occurs, your body starts breaking down existing structural proteins such as your muscles or connective tissue for the essential amino acids that it needs.

Essential Amino Acids
Histidine
Isoleucine
Leucine
Lysine
Methionine
Phenylalanine
Threonine
L-tryptophan
Valine

The nonessential amino acids are alanine, arginine, aspartic acid, asparagine, cysteine, glutamic acid, glutamine, glycine, proline, serine, and tyrosine. These amino acids are nonessential and nutritionally dispensable because your body can endogenously synthesize them from other essential amino acids or organic acids. However, nonessential amino acids are only nonessential if -- and only if -- you have enough of the essential amino acids or organic acids in order to synthesize them. This is an important point since it highlights the need for adequate daily protein intake. Eating enough protein daily will provide you with not only the essential amino acids but allow them to act as precursors for the nonessential amino acids synthesis. For example, the essential amino acid methionine and phenylalanine are precursors for the synthesis of the nonessential amino acids cysteine and tyrosine. Other non-essential amino acids are from organic acids, which is the combination of carbohydrates and nitrogen.

Non-essential Amino Acids
Alanine
Arginine
Aspartic Acid
Asparagine
Cysteine
Glutamic Acid
Glutamine
Glycine
Proline
Serine
Tyrosine

Amino acids that are nonessential at certain times may become "essential" at other times. The reason for this is due to your body's inability to synthesize enough of those nonessential amino acids to meet your body's demand. The other reason could stem from a deficiency of the essential amino acids due to a diet inadequate in daily protein intake. Cysteine, tyrosine, and glutamine are examples of nonessential amino acids that may not be synthesized in adequate amounts and that you are likely to be deficient in if you lack adequate protein. *Again, whenever there is an inadequate supply of the essential or nonessential amino acids for your body's metabolic needs, muscle and tissue protein breakdown occurs.*

The nutritional quality of a protein is measured by the efficiency with which the protein is able to meet your body's amino acids and nitrogen requirement – that is, its amino acid composition and its digestibility. A protein that is highly digestible and composed of a balanced pattern of amino acid is of higher quality then one that contains a disproportionately low amount of one or more amino acids or is incompletely digestible.

In 1993, the U.S. Food and Drug Administration (FDA) and the Food and Agricultural Organization of the United Nations (FAO), along with the World Health Organization (WHO), determined that the Protein Digestibility Corrected Amino Acid Score (PDCAAS) is the best method for evaluating the quality of the amino acid within a protein. A protein having a PDCAA score value of one is highest and a protein with a PDCAA score value of zero is the lowest. Examples of high quality protein sources are whey, milk, egg white, soy protein isolate and casein. Intermediate quality protein source are red meat, soybean, sunflower seed, rice, potato, and oats. Foods that are of low quality protein are peas, corn meal, and white flour.

All animal sources of proteins, such as red meat, chicken, pork, fish, milk, and eggs are complete proteins. A complete protein is one in which all the twenty amino acids are available during food ingestion. Yet a finer point to consider is the amount of the actual essential and nonessential amino acid within the protein. A food source that is a complete protein source does not tell you anything about the availability of the individual twenty amino acids found within the protein itself. It is due to this variability in the quantity of individual amino acid content within a protein source that makes getting an adequate amount of any specific essential or non-essential amino acid so unpredictable.

Given the unknown quantity of each amino acid within any given protein source, deficiencies of one amino acid over another can be magnified. As a rule to go by, one ounce of any red meat, chicken, pork, and fish has about seven grams of protein. A deck of card size serving, which is about three ounces, will have about twenty-one grams of protein.

The advantages of having enough protein for your body's daily needs are many. Protein intake is better for your metabolism. There is evidence that suggests protein increases thermogenesis, improve fat metabolism, and helps you eat less. When you are trying to cut calories, protein is the macronutrient needed since eating a higher protein meal tends to decrease appetite, enabling you to cut the carbohydrate calories. In addition, protein is the macronutrient needed to build muscle. This is an obvious statement for anyone that has tried to gain muscle mass. Less obvious, yet equally true, is what is good for your muscle must also be true for other organs in your body. You can consider your muscles as an organ just like your skin, heart, intestine, eyes, and brain. Individually these organs, along with many others, form a system you know as your body, and as such require adequate amounts of protein to function properly.

Lipids

Although the terms lipids and fats are sometimes used interchangeably, fats are a subgroup of lipids. Lipid is a broad term used to describe molecules such as fats, waxes, sterols such as cholesterol, fat-soluble vitamins and phospholipids. Lipid functions as a fuel source and as storable energy. In fact, lipids are the stored form of excessive calories. The adiposity (fatty tissue) that a person possesses is reflective of the abundance in consumed calories over his or her lifetime.

The amount of fats or lipids you should be eating daily, known as lipids RDA, varies from 20%-40% of your total daily caloric intake. In children age one to three years old, lipids' RDA is 30%-40%. For children age four to eighteen years old, the lipids' RDA is lower, at 25%-35%. For adults, the current lipids' RDA varies from 20%-35%.

Lipids are essential nutrients due to the role they serve in your body. The cells that you are composed of have an outer envelope made up of a bi-lipid layer, which is made of different phospholipids and cholesterol molecules. Cholesterols, a type of lipid, serve as precursors for important regulatory hormones such as cortisol and the sex hormones, estrogen and testosterone.

Different Types of Fats

Lipid is a term that encompasses different type of fat molecules. Fats are really fatty acid molecules and are composed of a chain of hydrocarbon linked together in a straight chain like fashion. A fatty acid molecule is saturated or unsaturated depending on how it exists in nature in the foods we eat. Fats are either solid (saturated fats) or liquid (unsaturated fats) at room temperature. Saturated and unsaturated fatty acids are formed from carbon atoms connected to each other in chains with a CH3 methyl group at one end. The methyl group end is the fat portion of the molecule and called the omega end. The other end of the carbon chain is connecting to a COOH carboxylic acid group. This carboxyl acid group end is the acid portion of the fatty acid. Saturated fatty acids are straight-line molecules consisting of carbon atoms connected to each other. The connections between the carbon atoms are single bonds with a hydrogen atom at the side-bonding site of the carbon chain. Since every bonding site on the carbon atom is filled with a hydrogen atom, the chain is saturated.

In addition, fatty acids are saturated or unsaturated fatty acids depending on whether they possess a double bond between the hydrocarbons. Unsaturated or essential fatty acids (EFA) will possess at least one double bond. A saturated fatty acid (SFA) or nonessential fatty acid will not possess any double bonds between the hydrocarbons. Unsaturated or essential fatty acids (EFA) and saturated fatty acid (SFA) are found in plant-based products (such as nuts and soybean) and in any animal-based foods product (such as meats). When we take an unsaturated fatty acid molecule and add an additional hydrogen atom molecule to it, it is now called a trans-fat. These trans-fatty acids do not exist in nature. Humans make trans-fatty acids by breaking the existing double bonds and adding additional hydrogen atoms. Trans-fatty acids are considered harmful for human health. According to the National Academy of Sciences, there is no safe level of consumption for trans-fatty acids. Two types of the unsaturated fatty acids that are crucial for health are omega-3 fatty acids and omega-6 fatty acids. The omega-3 EFA are named as such because the first double bond is at the third carbon-carbon bond from the omega end, which is the terminal CH3 end of the carbon chain. The omega-3 EFA are specifically the short chain polyunsaturated fatty acids (SC-PUFA), alpha-Linolenic acid or ALA. The long chain polyunsaturated fatty acids (LC-PUFA) are eicosapentaenoic acid (EPA) and docosahexaenoic acid (DHA). Part of the health benefits of the omega-3 LC-PUFA is based on their ability to decrease inflammation within our body. The omega-6 EFAs are called omega-6 fatty acids because the first double bond is at the sixth carbon- carbon bond from the omega end. The omega-6 EFAs are the linoleic acid (LA) and arachidonic acid. Since we cannot synthesize these unsaturated fatty acids, we have to consume them in our diet. (The saturated fatty acids, or SFAs, or nonessential fatty acids are not essential to our diet as we can make them from other nutrients such as proteins or carbohydrates.)

I believe that a deficiency in saturated fatty acid does not occur, even in individuals eating a low fat diet. The reason for this is that most of the foods consumed in a low fat diet will probably be low in fat content but are high in carbohydrates. With a low fat diet, deficiencies of saturated fatty acids and cholesterols will not occur, since if you did not consume any saturated fatty acid (SFA) or cholesterol from your diet, you are still able to synthesize saturated fatty acid and cholesterols. Your liver is able to synthesize SFA from carbohydrates. In fact, when you eat too many carbohydrates, your body is forced to convert these carbohydrate calories into fatty acids.

Lipids as nutrients and their role in health are misunderstood. People are told and believe that eating food high in fatty acids or lipids cause heart attacks and strokes. The association between hypercholesterolemia (high levels of cholesterol in the blood) and atherosclerosis (a condition in which fatty material collects on the walls of arteries) are touted by health experts, nutritional educators and by medical doctors. This is the reason for the traditional advice about eating a low fat diet as the key to keeping your blood lipids low. It is a mainstream belief that a low fat diet will result in a low blood lipid level and therefore translates to lowered cardiovascular risk factors. The assumption is that eating a diet high in fat causes hypercholesterolemia and this would then result in atherosclerosis. A low fat diet is believed to lower your cardiovascular risk by lowering your cholesterol level.

The fats or lipids that most individuals know about are the lipids discussed with them by their doctor when they have their cholesterols checked: total cholesterol, so-called "bad" cholesterol (LDL) and "good" cholesterol (HDL), along with triglycerides. It is believed that an individual's cholesterol level will correlate with his or her risk for cardiovascular diseases and stroke. The higher a person's blood cholesterol level, the higher the associated risk for diseases such as strokes and myocardial infarction (heart attack).

A person with a lower blood lipid level will have a lowered cardiovascular risk profile. Naturally, having a lowered lipid level is best. However, in my opinion, the best way to lower your blood lipid level is not by way of a low fat diet. In fact, this belief is misguided: A low fat diet pattern is the greatest risk factor for your high blood lipid level over time. This dietary pattern, with its intrinsic imbalance of macronutrients consumed, will actually raise your risk for cardiovascular diseases and stroke. In fact, a low fat diet does not do what the health experts claim. It does not lower your blood cholesterol level. Eating a low fat diet is precisely the reason you will have high blood levels of triglycerides (hypertriglyceridemia) and elevated blood fats, including cholesterol and triglycerides (hyperlipidemia). In my opinion, a low fat diet is the primary risk factor for the current obesity crisis in the United States.

Here's why: Your high blood lipid level is not due to the fatty foods you are eating. It is due to your own liver making those fats that is in your bloodstream – this process that we will discuss is known as liver de novo lipid genesis. Lipids are your body's main way to store excessive calories.

Let's take a closer look at this process. Each gram of fat provides 9 kcal per gram of energy. This means the amount of energy stored in fats is more than doubles the energy-storing capacity of either carbohydrates or proteins: Each of those only provides 4 kcal of potential energy per gram. When you overeat, the excessive calories – those consumed over the amount needed to support your metabolic demands -- are converted into fat by your liver. The conversion process of excessive calories into fat is the reason for the increased adiposity and waistline in over two-thirds of the individuals in the US population. Your body's metabolic processes are being hijacked to convert excessive calories into fats.

The question to ask is; "Why would your body want to make more cholesterol even when you are supposedly eating more than enough fat already?" The answer to this question is two-fold.

Your liver will produce the needed lipids when it perceives that there are deficiencies of lipids needed for health. From an evolutionary standpoint, the ability to make those nutrients needed in time of scarcity is a sure way to preserve the survival of that particular species. The second reason is simpler and it has to due with the amount of calories eaten. When you eat more calories than your body can use, your liver will convert those excessive calories into fats. The fats or lipid molecules will then travel through your bloodstream to get to their destination: the fat cells around your waistline. The precursor for the de novo synthesis of triglycerides and cholesterol is an abundance of calories consumed.

The excessive calories are usually due to an increase in carbohydrate intake, but they can also be from an excessive intake of proteins. The cholesterol results from your blood work will reflect your liver's endogenous cholesterol and triglyceride synthesis, which occurs any time excessive calories are consumed.

The drugs used to treat hypercholesterolemia are taken at nighttime because it is believed that most of your endogenous cholesterol synthesis occurs at nighttime. This method works because the medications are designed to inhibit endogenous cholesterol synthesis. This method of cholesterol lowering has nothing to do with inhibiting the fats that are absorbed from your diet. By inhibiting the endogenous production of cholesterols from your liver, your blood cholesterols levels are lowered.

Dietary intake of fats is not the major reason why an individual has high blood cholesterol (hypercholesterolemia). Why do most individuals have high blood cholesterol? The reasons are many but one answer is that in some cases, it is due to a genetic defect in the transport system of the LDL cholesterol molecule. However, I speculate that the major reason for hyperlipidemia is due to your body's increased synthesis of cholesterol. One reason this happens is due to you taking in more calories than your body needs. When this occurs, those calories are used, and those that are not used are stored as fats. Again, remember that what you eat or drink will be broken down into micronutrients and macronutrients consisting of lipids, carbohydrates, proteins, vitamins and minerals. Excessive calories eaten are not stored as proteins or to any considerable amount as sugars but as fats via your liver. Therefore, consuming a meal with too much carbohydrate will cause those calories to be first stored as glycogen, then fats. Fats are your body's long-term storage form for excessive calories.

A diet filled with food rich in carbohydrate has two potential adverse effects. The first one is that this diet is imbalanced and will lack the proper amount of needed proteins. The second adverse affect is that the excessive carbohydrates eaten will stimulate the release of insulin. Insulin release promotes the storage of consumed carbohydrate calories as fats. The fat that is produced by the liver will eventually be stored in adipose tissue. However, before it is stored in your adipose tissue, it needs to travel in one's bloodstream. Therefore, when looking at the results of a blood cholesterol test, the high blood cholesterols seen could be reflective of a diet high in excessive carbohydrates. The increased adiposity and obesity with resultant high blood cholesterol is really the result of a diet with excessive carbohydrate calories intake.

For individuals with high blood cholesterol, the current dietary recommendation is to avoid food high in fat such as red meat. This recommendation can help to lower a person's blood cholesterol level if dietary fat intake is the sole cause for a person to have high blood cholesterol. But the recommendation to avoid red meat is putting individuals at greater risk of protein deficiency. Moreover, they can still have high cholesterol since the avoidance of the fat within red meat is not the full story regarding high blood cholesterol. The other part of the story is too much carbohydrate intake.

The more important question to ask here is, "Are there other causes for atherosclerosis beside excessive carbohydrate consumption that drives the liver to produce too many fats – or in doctor speak, that result in endogenous hypercholesterolemia synthesis?" I believe that there are. I suggest that the deficiencies of proteins and vitamin D can also play a role for the increased production of lipids. I will address these points later in the discussion for the causes of cardiovascular diseases and vitamin D deficiency.

Vitamins and Minerals

Classified as micronutrients, vitamins and minerals are essential for good health. You need micronutrients daily and their availability is essential. Unlike the macronutrients, your body does not have the capacity to store any excessive amounts of micronutrients consumed from a given meal. Micronutrients consumed are either used or excreted. The amount of a particular vitamin or mineral needed depends on one's daily metabolic demands. Fat-soluble vitamins are an exception since they can be stored in your adipose tissues when consumed in excessive amounts. Yet over time, deficiencies in daily intake will deplete these storable forms and the stored fat-soluble vitamins can no longer meet your needs.

The role that vitamins and minerals play in your health depends on the specific amounts of vitamins or minerals consumed. The likelihood that you are deficient in any specific vitamin or mineral will depend on the foods you choose to eat daily. *The beneficial health affects from eating foods such as fruits or vegetables are due to the vitamins, minerals and antioxidant properties that they contain.*

The beneficial health affects from eating fruits and vegetables, with their abundance of vitamins and minerals, are endless, especially since the over-consumption and toxicity from the vitamins and minerals in foods are extremely rare. Your body has the mechanism for dealing with the over-consumption of micronutrients that is uniquely different then the overconsumption of macronutrients.

The over-consumption of macronutrient leads your body to store the unused macronutrient calories as fats. As for micronutrients, your body is able to self regulate the amount of needed vitamins and minerals consumed daily and, with the exception of the fat soluble vitamins A, D, E and K, will excrete what it does not need. However, eating too many fruits and vegetables can still lead to an over-consumption of sugar calories and this, so far, has not been pointed out. Since most Americans eat too few fruits, this may not be a concern. However, the most consumed vegetables are potatoes, corn and corn by products (all are high in carbohydrates).

Although most people consider peas and beans to be vegetables, they are technically legumes and are fruits belonging to the family Leguminosae or. Fabaceae Examples of well-known legumes are alfalfa, clover, peas, beans, lupines, mesquite, carob and peanuts. Legumes are a food often used by vegetarians as their source of protein. They are an incomplete source of protein and will need to be combined with another food source in order to make them become a complete protein.

The colors of fruits and vegetables are beneficial due to plant chemicals that create them and their antioxidant properties. Consider antioxidants as those vitamins and minerals that help the body get rid of free radicals produced during the normal process of cell repair, replacement, or maintenance. Free radicals are the by-product of normal cellular metabolism. Antioxidants help protect the cell from the damaging effects of free radicals. Free radicals damage your cells in a way similar to how "electrostatic energy" can short circuit an electronic circuit board.

There are published guidelines as to the amounts of vitamins and minerals that an adult should take daily. Within most multivitamins, the amounts of vitamins or minerals are represented as a percentage of the recommended daily allowance (RDA). The RDA for most vitamins or minerals found in multivitamins; however, does not represent the amount needed for optimal health. The reason for this is that the RDA is really the minimal amount that has been determined to prevent an illness or disease from happening and not for optimal health.

An example would be vitamin C. The RDA for vitamin C is currently only 67 mg per day. A deficiency in vitamin C causes scurvy, a disease that occurs due to the lack of collagen synthesis. A daily dose of 67 mg per day of vitamin C is supposed to prevent a person from getting scurvy. Therefore, 67 mg of vitamin C is the amount needed daily and is the current 100% RDA for vitamin C. However, I believe that this dose is considerably less than the optimal amount needed for optimal health. Vitamin C is an antioxidant and as such, the actual amount needed is a greater amount than the current RDA.

Another vitamin recommended at an inadequate amount is vitamin D. The current RDA for vitamin D is only 600 IU (international units) per day for an adult. The upper limit advisable for vitamin D, without any adverse effects from vitamin D toxicity, is 4000 IU per day. There are existing studies that concluded that this amount is inadequate as the actual amount needed may be up to 10,000 IU for some individuals.

Vitamin D is widely thought of as the sunshine vitamin because our body is able to make vitamin D from the sun's ultraviolet B (UV-B) light. The truth about vitamin D is that most people work indoors, in a nine to five job; they and other people who are housebound are almost certainly vitamin D deficient. The prevalence of vitamin D deficiency affects up to

80% of U.S. adults. In the New England Journal of Medicine, Michael F. Holick, M.D., Ph.D., presented a review article in which he referenced the wide range of conditions associated with vitamin D deficiency, including cardiovascular disease, diabetes mellitus, multiple sclerosis, and cancer. From a meta-analysis of 18 randomized, controlled trials of the use of vitamin D supplementation, researchers concluded that individuals randomly assigned to take supplemental vitamin D had a statistically significant 7% reduction in mortality from any cause.

Except for vitamin D's current use in maintaining bone health, its broad health potential continues to be underutilized. I believe that it is such an important micronutrient that it deserves a separate discussion in itself. Therefore, I would like to take a moment to discuss more fully the role that vitamin D deficiency plays in human health. I will also give specific physiological evidence as to why vitamin D deficiency is the cause for diseases like osteoporosis and impaired fasting glucose, or a term that more people may come to hear more of: "insulin resistance."

In the next chapter, I will discuss the clinical significance of vitamin D deficiency in context of its role in the regulation of calcium homeostasis and in its lesser-known role as a nuclear receptor signal. In addition, I will give examples of the potential adverse effects caused by vitamin D deficiency in patients who are on commonly used medications such as cholesterol lowering drugs or certain cardiac medications.

Vitamin D

Fat-soluble vitamins abound if you consume fats from animals. From an evolutionary perspective, fat-soluble vitamins are an ingenious way to conserve essential vitamin nutrients needed during time of scarcity. Nevertheless, this assumption only holds if you have an adequate amount of the fat-soluble vitamins already stored for time of scarcity. This is not always the case for vitamin D. Vitamin D is a fat-soluble vitamin and when a deficiency occurs, it will take time for it to be corrected since your fat stores are depleted. (Micronutrients such as minerals and most vitamins, in contrast, are not stored for times of scarcity. Water-soluble vitamins consumed in excess are excreted through the kidney or gut.)

Vitamin D deficiency is very prevalent. Clinically, about 90% of the patients I see are either vitamin D insufficient or deficient. This means that their blood serum vitamin D 25-OH level is less than the level that is currently determined to be optimal for health. The detection of vitamin D deficiency is by a blood test of the 25-hydroxy vitamin D level. (The exact value for the lower limit of vitamin D varies depending on the laboratory used.) According to Dr. Michael Holick, a medical expert on vitamin D, a value of 32 ng/ml is the lower threshold for optimal health. A level above this would help protect against secondary hyperparathyroidism and its resulting ills.

I believe a vitamin D 25-OH of less then 32 ng/dl is harmful. The level of vitamin D 25-OH thought to be optimal is unknown. Nevertheless, I believe it should be at least 70 ng/dl. With all my patients, I make it a priority to discuss the high prevalence of vitamin D deficiency and the need to treat the deficiency.

One of the most common questions that I get after patients discover that they are either vitamin D insufficient or deficient is, "Why is my vitamin D level so low?" In other words, "Why is vitamin D deficiency so prevalent?" The simple answer to this question is that most individuals are not outside in the sunlight at the time of day needed for vitamin D synthesis.

We obtain vitamin D from two sources. The first is the synthesis of vitamin D from UV-B sunlight exposure and the second is from the foods that we eat. From a dietary standpoint, very few natural foods have vitamin D. Some foods that do, include fatty fish, cod liver oil, and egg yolk. I am sometimes pleasantly surprised that cod liver oil is what some of my patients took when they were children. I find that foods alone are a poor source for vitamin D since an individual's daily requirement of vitamin D is much higher than what foods can generally provide. Thus, in order to have an adequate amount of vitamin D daily, artificially supplementing vitamin D instead of more exposure of UV-B sunlight exposure is my preferred treatment option.

Synthesis of vitamin D

We are able to synthesize vitamin D from the UV-B light shining on our skin. Vitamin D synthesis occurs at the two inner layer of our epidermis.

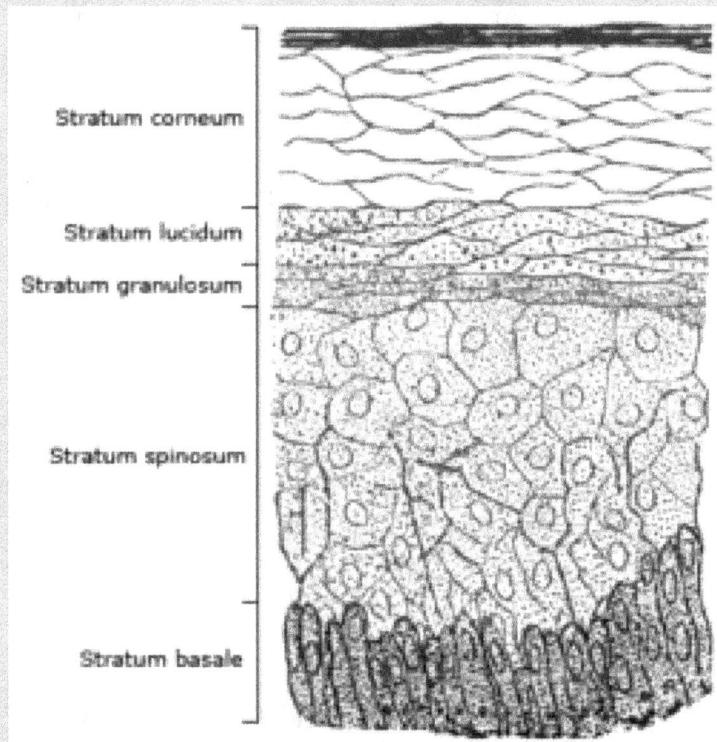

The epidermal strata of the skin. Vitamin D production is greatest in the stratum basale (bottom layer) and stratum spinosum (thickest layer).

http://en.wikipedia.org/wiki/File:Skinlayers.png

The amount of sunlight exposure needed for vitamin D synthesis is about 10 to 15 minutes to the skin of our face, hands, or back. The sunlight exposure needs to be direct sunlight contact on the skin surface and not exposure through a glass window, car window or skin coated with suntan lotion. Windows and suntan lotion will make the sunlight ineffective for the synthesis of vitamin D. In addition, if you are a dark skinned individual or an older adult, you will produce less vitamin D from any sun exposure, even if you have sufficient UV-B exposure.

The synthesis of vitamin D is a multi-step process requiring the penetration of the skin by UV-B radiation exposure. When this happens, a chain reaction activates the liver and kidney to produce the active 1-25 OH vitamin D molecule. Any disruption or dysfunction in this multi-step processes can account for you being vitamin D deficient. The ultraviolet UV-B radiation needed to activate the process of vitamin D synthesis is when the sun is at 45 degrees above the horizon for a person living at sea level. The optimal time of the day that would correspond to 45 degrees above the horizon is the period between 10 am to about 4 pm in the afternoon.

Other factors that affect UV-B radiation roles on vitamin D synthesis have to do with where a person lives relative to the equator. The wavelength of ultraviolet B radiation that is effective for vitamin D synthesis is anything below the 35 degrees north of the equator. Individuals living north of 37 degrees of the equator -- roughly a line drawn from Richmond, Virginia to San Francisco will reveal regions that do not have any vitamin D synthesis from November through February regardless of the duration of sunlight exposure. People living between 30 to 35 degrees latitude, including New Mexico and most of Texas have insufficient UVB sunlight for two months out of the year.

Vitamin D is called a vitamin but it actually functions as a hormone. It is synthesized from a cholesterol molecule and has hormonal and gene regulatory function. Ultraviolet B radiation exposure on your skin activates vitamin D synthesis. You need an adequate amount of vitamin D every day for specific cellular function. If you are outside at the right time of day for ultraviolet B exposure to activate vitamin D synthesis, your body will have more than enough vitamin D for the day. If the vitamin D made for the day is not used, then your body has the capacity to store the excess amounts in your adipose tissue.

When you are not getting adequate daily sunlight exposure, your body will not have an adequate amount of vitamin D needed for your body's metabolic demands. The consequences from the inability to synthesize enough vitamin D for a day or for a short time period will not have clinical significance since your body has stored excessive vitamin D in your adipose tissue. Over time, however, because of your body's inadequate daily vitamin D synthesis, you will deplete the vitamin D stored in your adipose tissue. The depleted vitamin D in your adipose tissue is the first-step of multiple steps toward the harmful health effects of vitamin D deficiency.

Adverse Affects of vitamin D Deficiency
1. Hypocalcemia (low calcium levels) with secondary hyperparathyroidism
2. Impairment of the gene regulatory function

The adverse affects of vitamin D deficiency are two fold. The first is through vitamin D's role in calcium regulation. The active form of vitamin D, the 1, 25-dihydroxyvitamin D3, is integral to calcium homeostasis (equilibrium). The 1, 25-dihydroxyvitamin D3 acts on the intestine, kidneys, and bones, regulating calcium homeostasis. Moreover, evidence indicates the presence of the 1, 25-dihydroxyvitamin D3 receptors in nearly every type of cell in the body. A deficiency in the active 1, 25-dihydroxyvitamin D3 potentially can affect calcium balance at each individual cell, potentially leading to a "relative" hypocalcemia (abnormally low calcium levels in the blood). The active form of vitamin D is also important for regulating dietary calcium absorption.

Vitamin D deficiency has a stimulatory effect on your parathyroid gland leading to secondary hyperparathyroidism (an enlargement of one or more of the parathyroid glands, which causes overproduction of the hormone that results in high levels of calcium in the blood). The adverse health effect of vitamin D deficiency is from the abnormally low calcium levels (hypocalcemia) as the result of the deficiency and the secondary hyperparathyroidism that resulted from the onset of hypocalcemia.

The second adverse effect of vitamin D deficiency is through vitamin D's role in gene regulation. The active 1-25 OH vitamin D molecule, as you may remember, is involved in gene regulation. In discussing vitamin D's role in gene regulation, I will explain how impairment of the gene regulatory function of the active vitamin D is a possible cause for insulin resistance, impaired fasting glucose, and obesity.

Without active vitamin D acting on the gut, the absorption of calcium in the gut is inhibited. The decreased gut absorption of calcium will result in a hypocalcemic state. However, before hypocalcemia can fully occur, your body will secrete parathyroid hormone. Secondary hyperparathyroidism will then initiate your bone osteoclasts (bone-reabsorbing cells) to begin breaking down your bone for the needed calcium.

But here's the kicker: Even when severe vitamin D deficiency exists, your blood serum calcium value will be normal. The reason for this is that secondary hyperparathyroidism will act on your skeleton since it is your body's natural reservoir for calcium.

In clinical practice, the cause and effect between vitamin D deficiency and osteoporosis is not recognized. In fact, if one were to look at the top five risk factors for osteoporosis, I can tell you that vitamin D deficiency is not on that list. I believe that vitamin D deficiency is more that just a risk factor but the actual cause for osteopenia and osteoporosis. In fact, vitamin D deficiency may be the cause of a lot of the "age"-related degenerative musculoskeletal disease that we get as we become older.

For this reason, once osteoporosis is diagnosed, the first test that should be obtained (after a bone density scan that has revealed bone loss) is the patient's vitamin D level. Yet clinically I see that this test is rarely performed. Instead, patients are customarily advised to take supplemental calcium with added vitamin D and, if deemed appropriate by their doctor, bisphosphonates. While this recommendation is the norm, it neglects the need to detect and treat the primary defect -- or as I would like to think about it, the root cause -- a vitamin D deficiency. Addressing the vitamin D deficiency would most likely result in a greater improvement in bone density. This is because without adequate active vitamin D, the calcium consumed will not be absorbed adequately.

The current recommended daily allowance (RDA) of vitamin D is only 600 IU a day for an adult. This amount is severely inadequate for most adults and especially those that are already showing evidence of osteopenia or osteoporosis. Most osteopenia and osteoporotic individuals are probably taking too little vitamin D to correct the vitamin D deficiency that exists. The reason for this is that the dose of vitamin D that those individuals are taking every day is not even enough to fulfill their daily maintenance requirement dose, let alone address an existing deficiency.

One of the top five risk factors for osteopenia (bone mineral density that is lower than normal) and osteoporosis is genetic because both seem to run in a person's family. For example, if you have osteoporosis and your mother and grandmother both has osteoporosis, chances are you are told that osteoporosis "runs in your family." To say that an illness or disease runs in a person's family is to imply that it is inheritable. I believe that genetics is not the reason why osteoporosis generally occurs. The lack of recognition of vitamin D deficiency and its health effects has made a disease like osteoporosis seem like it is genetically determined. On the contrary, I believe osteoporosis is not inherited but manifests through the effects of vitamin D deficiency. It is due to the lack of the active vitamin D needed for proper calcium regulation.

The use of bisphosphonates for patients with osteoporosis is common. In clinical practice, bisphosphonates are a class of prescription medication used for the treatment of osteoporosis. A common symptom experienced in individuals using one of the bisphosphonates is joint pain (arthralgia) and even osteonecrosis (death of bone tissue). I believe arthralgia and osteonecrosis are due to an aggravation of the effects of vitamin D deficiency by the use of bisphosphonates. Since bisphosphonates work to inhibit the actions of osteoclasts, this medication can worsen the hypocalcemia that already exists in a patient with vitamin D deficiency. Hypocalcemia, as we've discussed, leads to secondary hyperparathyroidism. Secondary hyperparathyroidism causes osteomalacia (a softening of the bone) and shows up as diffuse skeletal pain and proximal muscle weakness. The radiographic finding of patients with osteomalacia shows a bone mineral density that is lower than normal (osteopenia).

The possibility of severe, sometimes debilitating bone, joint, and/or musculoskeletal pain in patients taking bisphosphonates was made known in a FDA alert notice letter that went out on 1/7/2008 to physicians; on November 30, 2010, the FDA sent another letter warning doctors that cancer patients taking certain bisphosphonates were at higher risk of developing death of the jawbone (osteonecrosis of the jaw). The problem with this type of alert letter is that physicians are still unaware of the implications of this warning regarding the bisphosphonates class of anti-osteoporosis drugs.

In a vitamin D deficient state, your body's calcium requirement often exceeds calcium availability. When this occurs, your body attempts to maintain a normal serum calcium level via secondary hyperparathyroidism. However, as secondary hyperparathyroidism tries to correct a relative hypocalcemia state, an unintended transient high calcium and high phosphate level can result. The detrimental health effect from a high calcium/ high phosphate level is not often recognized as being caused by vitamin D deficiency. Patients with hyperparathyroidism, renal (kidney) failure, and those on dialysis frequently exhibit a high presence of hydroxyapatite, a mineral primarily found in bone and teeth. Similarly, hydroxyapatite is in the joint fluid of 50% of patients with osteoarthritis. I believe that secondary hyperparathyroidism resulting from a vitamin D deficiency can cause the condition known as osteoarthritis.

Other signs and symptoms of secondary hyperparathyroidism include gastrointestinal manifestations, such as vague abdominal pains and disorders of the stomach. Increased stomach acid may be present with heartburn, gastritis, or ulcers. The success of acid-inhibiting medications, such as H2 blockers or PPI's, in helping patients with increased acid disease live symptom-free are undeniable. However, patients often experience a reappearance of symptoms upon stopping these medications. Some of these patients therefore require continuous use of an acid-suppressing medication for indefinite lengths of time. The link between secondary hyperparathyroidism and gastrointestinal symptoms suggests an imbalance in calcium metabolism as a potential basis for heartburn, gastritis, and/or ulcers.

Another adverse effect of secondary hyperparathyroidism from vitamin D deficiency that can be seen, but often remain unrecognized, is cardiovascular disease, such as hypertension and, specifically, arterial calcification. Calciphylaxis is a syndrome of tissue necrosis (death) resulting from arterial calcification. Patients with end-stage renal disease who are undergoing hemodialysis often have calciphylaxis. The pathogenesis of calciphylaxis is unclear, but two associated risk factors are hyperparathyroidism and an elevated calcium-phosphorus product. As we age, arterial vascular calcification is common. The conventional teaching is that the etiology of arterial vascular calcification associated with aging is secondary to high blood fat levels (hyperlipidemia), and the arterial calcification due to high blood fat levels is atherosclerosis. However, in the life of an individual with vitamin D deficiency, one might ask, "Could arterial calcification result in some degree not from high blood fats, but from the same risk factors as calciphylaxis?"

Elevated calcium-phosphorus product is not typically a condition associated with secondary hyperparathyroidism, unless there is kidney dysfunction and tertiary hyperparathyroidism. However, can a severe vitamin D deficiency state present in a similar picture? My theory is that osteoarthritis, osteoporosis, GERD, and hypertension can be linked directly to a vitamin D deficiency via secondary hyperparathyroidism.

Medication and Vitamin D Deficiency

In a vitamin D deficient patient, certain medications should be used with caution. As previously discussed, bisphosphonates use may worsen hypocalcemia and cause musculoskeletal pains and joint symptoms in a vitamin D deficient patient. Such potentially avoidable side effects associated with the use of certain medications in a vitamin D deficient state extends to other drugs, as well -- namely, those belonging to the class of medication called "statins."

The tendency for certain cholesterol-lowering drugs to cause side effects such as myopathy (muscle disease not due to a nerve disorder), abnormal liver function, and rhabdomyolysis (the rapid, potentially fatal breakdown of skeletal muscle due to injury to muscle tissue) are often attributed to the way these medications are metabolized via the liver cytochrome P450 enzyme system -- specifically, the metabolism by the specific CYP3A4 enzyme. Medications that fall into this category, called "statins," are associated with a risk of myalgia (muscle pain), hepatotoxicity (chemical-driven liver damage), and rhabdomyolysis.

In the presence of competing substances that use the same cytochrome P450 pathway, the breakdown of one of these drugs is inhibited. This interference creates a risk of prolonging the effects or increasing the level of the medication. For example, grapefruit juice consumption by a patient taking 80 mg of lovastatin or 60 mg of simvastatin a day results in a 15-fold increase in drug level. A higher level of these cholesterol-lowering drugs should translate to a greater ability for this drug to inhibit cholesterol synthesis. A greater ability to inhibit cholesterol synthesis may not be a desirable result, as cholesterol is integral to bile acid synthesis and serves as a precursor for vitamin D synthesis.

Statins can affect vitamin D level through a lower bile acid level and lower cholesterol as a vitamin D precursor. The greater the decrease in bile acid, the lower the chance that dietary vitamin D will supplement a deficiency that already existed at baseline. Thus, statins can cause an even greater deficiency, thus leading to the symptoms associated with severe lack of active 1, 25-dihydroxyvitamin D3. Hypocalcemia causes myopathy (muscle disease); hyperphosphatemia (an increased concentration of inorganic phosphates in the blood) from secondary hyperparathyroidism can cause rhabdomyolysis (the rapid destruction of skeletal muscle). The consequences of vitamin D deficiency explain the side effects associated with these cholesterol-lowering drugs.

Another way cholesterol-lowering drugs can affect vitamin D levels is by inhibiting the bile acid synthesis itself through the inhibition of a subfamily of the cytochrome P450 system, CYP27, which is responsible for bile acid synthesis. Other known drug-to-drug, drug-to-food, or drug-to-fluid intake interactions, such as QT-prolongations, are due to alteration of calcium homeostasis.

Vitamin D deficiency is startlingly common. In this chapter, I have attempted to shed light on the mechanisms of the effects of vitamin D deficiency on bone health, and will explore its possible link to obesity, high blood fats and insulin resistance in subsequent chapters. The information on hypocalcemia and secondary hyperparathyroidism is factual. My presentation of the mechanism of known, adverse side effects with certain medications is related to knowledge of the consequences of vitamin D deficiency, specifically the alteration of calcium homeostasis.

My goal of emphasizing the health effects of vitamin D is to highlight the overlooked associations between vitamin D deficiency and other medical illnesses and diseases. Obviously, treating this key vitamin deficiency could not only result in improved health, but might help ward off a host of debilitating chronic diseases.

The Cell

In trying to understand how nutrition affects your health, it is important to understand how the human cell works. I will only touch on some basic information so that you can appreciate the wonders of it. Believe me when I say that a complete understanding of a single human cell would be the first step to understanding the complexities of the human body. Small wonder that I do not claim to understand completely the workings within the human cell.

When you look in the mirror, the reflected image you see of yourself is of a highly complex organized meshwork of cells. These cells all fit together to give a physical image you recognize as yourself. If you analyze what you are composed of under a high power microscope, the answer would be cells. All of us are composed of about an estimated 10 trillion cells. In a lifetime, the average human being goes through about 10^{16} cell divisions. Every day there are about 10^{11} cells that divide and grow daily. The largest human cell is about 100 microns in diameter. A cell 100 microns in diameter is about as thick as a human hair.

Most human cells are much smaller then the diameter of a human hair and is perhaps only one-tenth of the diameter of your hair (10 microns). To give a little perspective on the number of cells there are in our body -- an estimated 10 trillion cells -- here is an example. A trillion is 1000 billion. There are about two or three billion cells in your little toe.

Everything from the time of your conception to death happens down at the cellular level. Your cells are called eukaryotes. A eukaryotic cell is a cell that has a nucleus that is surrounded by its own membrane. (This is different than the prokaryotic cell such as a bacteria cell. A prokaryotic cell does not have a membrane surrounding its nuclear material. A prokaryotic cell also lacks other important cellular structure found in a eukaryotic cell.) When one or more of the eukaryotic cells come together, they now form multi-cellular cells. Multi-cellular cells include epithelia cells, connective tissue cells, muscle cells, and lastly neuronal cells. These different types of cells all serve as a vital part in forming a higher organizational system from a single cell to tissues, to organs, and then organ systems.

Cells that form multi-cellular cells are derived from the differentiation of multi-potent stem cells. Stem cells can differentiate into about 200 different cell types. Some examples of what stem cells can transform into include muscle cells, skin cells, bone cells and neuronal cells.

A cell is composed of an outer envelope called the cell membrane. This cell membrane is formed from phospholipids, proteins and cholesterol molecules. The membrane separates what is considered outside the cell versus the inside content of the cell.

Within the cell membrane lies a fluid called the cytoplasm. The cytoplasm is composed of about 70% water, with the other 30% being organelles and proteins. Water is an important nutrient needed for life because of its central role in many of the metabolic reactions needed for life. In order for cellular reaction to occur, water often is central or a by-product of that metabolic reaction. Water is used for the formation of peptide bonds, which are used to hold amino acids together in a protein. A chemical reaction where water is the by-product is in the Krebs cycle (the common pathway to oxidize fuel molecules). In the conversion of glucose in your body to usable energy of ATP in the Krebs cycle, water molecules are formed.

At any given moment, different enzymes are doing work inside the cells of your body. Understanding of the diverse function of enzymes is critical to understanding the cell. The bacteria E. coli, has about 1,000 different types of enzymes in its cytoplasm. The enzymes play a diverse function in the cells, such as assisting in metabolic reaction. The purpose of a cell's enzyme is to allow the cell to carry out multiple chemical reactions very quickly. Enzymes, in fact, are proteins that enable chemical reactions to occur at a faster rate then otherwise possible. Without help from enzymes, certain chemical reactions would not occur in the first place. The chemical reactions that enzymes carry out enable the cell to synthesize new molecules or to break down existing molecules. This is how a cell is able to grow and reproduce.

Although enzymes are proteins, they are, more specifically, chains of amino acids. Amino acids are the basic buildings block that makes up proteins. A protein is the linkage of a string of between hundreds to thousands of amino acids linked together by peptide bonds. Each protein has a specific, unique characteristic depending on the sequences of the amino acids. A protein can fold into unique shapes depending on how the amino acid chain is sequenced. Each protein with its unique shape allows it to function as an enzyme carrying out specific chemical reactions. Perhaps the best way to put it is this: Enzymes are the catalyst for specific chemical reactions, so that the speed of a reaction occurs efficiently and at a faster rate than otherwise possible.

Your genetic code or DNA determines the arrangements of the sequences of amino acids. The syntheses of any enzymes needed in your body are dependent on their function and probably secondarily, the availability of the different amino acids within the enzymes. The aspect of not having a specific amino acid required for the synthesis of a protein may not have been considered. Clinically, deficiencies of the amino acids required for protein synthesis will not be noticed as a relative inability to make a certain enzyme. In real life, situations like the one just described will occur and if they become chronic, present as susceptibility for illnesses or as a disease.

Amino acids are the small molecules that act as the building blocks of any protein. Without the correct amino acids or the amounts needed, protein syntheses are restricted and limited. This fact has a direct effect on the health and well-being of your body.

At the center of the cell is a membrane-bound material called the nucleus. The nucleus carries the genes of the cell, and it is the genetic material that is the blueprint of who you are. Every one of your 10 trillion cells has a nucleus containing this blueprint. The nucleus contains the instructions for every cell function in your body. The nucleus also has the instructions that will govern the life span of that individual cell. The instructions for when a cell will divide and when it will stop dividing and undergo cell death, called apoptosis, are in the nucleus.

All the codes, for the synthesis of the different enzymes needed for life, lie in the cell nucleus or its DNA (deoxyribonucleic acid). Your DNA is the genetic material that codes for all the proteins needed for life. It is composed of chain of nucleotide acids, similar to the amino acids that compose a protein. The DNA in your cells is composed of four nucleotides or bases. Imagine that your genes are composed of an alphabet that has only four different letters. These nucleotides code for the message needed for a cell to make protein and other cellular function such as cell division.

A prokaryotic cell such as an E. coli cell has DNA the size that is about four million nucleotides long. If you were to stretch out the DNA of an E. coli, this single stand of DNA would be approximately 1.36 mm long. This length is considerably longer then the bacteria itself -- by about 1,000 times. Within the bacteria cell, the bacteria DNA strand is wadded up like a ball of string. A human's nucleus DNA strand is about 3 billion nucleotides long, or almost 1,000 times longer than that of an E. coli. A human DNA strand is longer then a bacterium and cannot be wadded up into a ball of string like a bacterium. However, instead of organizing your DNA like a ball of string, the human DNA is a double helical pattern, like that of a ladder. In addition, to make the length of your genes "manageable," the double helix is not a single long strand but cut into 23 structural lengths called chromosomes. This arrangement enables the human cell's DNA to be packed tightly into the cell's nucleus.

Your brain is made of approximately 100-billion nerve cells, called neurons. These neurons are able to receive and transmit electrochemical signals. Every neuron shares the same characteristics and has the same parts as any other cells in your body. In fact, the parts that make up your neurons are probably the same as in any other animals that live on this earth. What distinguishes your neurons from the other cells in your body are 1) the length of the neuronal cells and 2) the life span of the neuronal cells. These differences distinguish them from other cell types in your body.

A neuron has three basic parts: a cell body, an axon, and dendrites or nerve endings. The cell body is the part that has all of the necessary components of the cell, such as the nucleus (which contains DNA), endoplasmic reticulum and ribosome (for building proteins) and mitochondria (for making energy). The axon is the long cable-like projection from the cell body that carries electrochemical messages as nerve impulses or action potential along the length of the cell.

Depending upon the type of neuron, the axons are covered with a thin layer of myelin, similar to the insulated plastic around an electrical wire. Myelin is made of fat molecules such as cholesterol and the omega 3 fatty acids. Myelin helps speed the transmission of a nerve impulse down the long axon. Myelinated neurons are typically found in the peripheral nerves (sensory and motor neurons), while non-myelinated neurons are found in the brain and spinal cord.

Dendrites or nerve endings are small, branch-like projections from the cell body that connect one neuronal cell to another neuronal cell. This allows many neurons to talk with each other or to perceive the environment. Dendrites are located on one or both ends of the cell body. The brain neuron in some ways is "hard-wired" with connections, much as how a computer or house is hard-wired by electrical wiring. In the case of the brain, the connections are by neurons that connect the sensory inputs and motor outputs with centers in the various lobes of the cortex. There are also connections between these cortical centers and other parts of the brain.

Apoptosis is a biological term used to refer to cell death. A cell can die in one of the three ways. The first is through programmed cell death. The second is by necrosis -- the premature death of cells and living tissue -- due to ischemia (a restriction in blood supply). The third is due to autophagy (a process that occurs when cells confront an inadequate supply of nutrients in their extracellular fluid and may start to cannibalize some of their internal organelles such as mitochondria). When the normal cell cycle regulation is lost, a cell is able to grow out of control and may become a cancer cell. Therefore, the normal processes of life are that of cell differentiation, cell division and cell death. These processes take place over and over, from the time of initial fertilization of a spermatocyte and oocyte to the time of death of the individual. What this means is that even though you function as a complex multi-cellular individual that might look the same on the outside; your cells are constantly undergoing changes not perceived by you. Some of the changes occurring to your cells daily are cell repair, cell replacement or cell death.

From the information discussed, you must now know that some of the cells that you are composed of today are likely not the same cells you had yesterday, and are especially unlikely to be the same cells you had at birth. The reason is that a tremendous number of cells turn over daily. Remember that every day, there are about 10^{11} cells that grow and divide daily. These turnovers of cells happen for a reason -- growth, development and aging. The fuel for the growth and development of cells are from the food nutrients you consume. This is why the food nutrients you consume play such a critical role in your health. *Deficiencies of micronutrients and macronutrients needed versus that actually consumed daily could be the very reason we have illnesses and chronic diseases*.

Protein's Link to Brain Information Storage: A Theory

The following information that I am about to discuss next is very theoretical. It is hypothetical since I am trying to understand and explain a process that no one really understands. To wit: Information taken in by your eyes needs to be processed and stored in some manner. How your brain processes the information is unknown, much less how the information is stored. Still, I will attempt to speculate how information is stored in your brain. If we compare your eyes to a movie camera, then all the pictures taken through your eyes from the time you are born to the time you die will need to be stored on some type of medium for retrieval. The storage and retrieval of these pictures are easier to think about in terms of "films" in a camera. Camera film in a digital age is no longer film but data on memory sticks or cards.

In order for something to be retrievable, it must first be stored in a way that is lasting or permanent. From a biological standpoint, unlike a film, memory disk or chip, the question of how a living cell is able to achieve this goal needs discovering. It is believed that all your cells have a finite lifespan. The exceptions to this lifespan are neuronal (nerve) cells, which are believed to have a longer lifespan. This means that neuronal cells can store information that has the potential to be "permanent." Brain cells --whether neuronal cells or non-neuronal -- support cells call glial cells needed to store information in a form that is not only permanent but accurate and retrievable. The information stored needs to be retrievable for later use. However, before information can be retrieved, it has to be "written" in some form in your brain. Think of how you go about writing down information you want to recall later in time. You can write it on a chalkboard, a piece of paper, or type it on a computer where that information will be stored as bits of information using 1's and O's on a memory circuit board. Could your brain use a technique similar to a computer to store information?

The question to ask next is, "Where and how do you store the information that is taken in every day?" The thing that has always struck me as amazing is how similar your brain could be to a computer. A computer is able to store information on a circuit board consisting of memory chips. The memory chips contain transistors that hold electrical charges as 1 or 0. The 1 and 0 represent an electrical current on the transistor of the memory chip as being either charged or not charged. Therefore the 1 and 0 is the binary language that a computer uses to store data. For your brain, could the comparable 1 and 0 be in the form of proteins or amino acids helping neuronal cells store information?

I believe the proteins found in the neuronal cells of your brain can act as data storage similar to the 1 and O of a transistor of a memory chip. Proteins play a critical role in almost every aspect of cellular function. As such, the possibility that proteins are what your body uses to store information may not be impossible. The possibility that neuronal cells play a role in storing data as proteins is likely, since proteins possess intrinsic charges. Each protein structure possesses charges that can function similar to the 1 and O on a memory chips. In fact, if proteins were indeed what your brain used to store information, this theory would explain the causes for Alzheimer's.

The possibility that proteins serve as memory chips does pose some problems. In order for your brain to use proteins to code information, proteins must always be available. In addition, because proteins may not be stable indefinitely, there must be a mechanism to ensure the stability of the proteins. This requires that the information that the protein encodes be permanent so that the information is retrievable at any time. In order for proteins to function in memory, they must be able to be replicated if needed.

"So how might they be replicated? Let's consider the cell's DNA. The cell's DNA functions as the blueprint for life. Your DNA is the actual blueprint that your body uses to make the proteins that act as enzymes and other structural proteins. Without proteins, life as we know it would not exist. Francis Crick delineated the pathway of DNA to protein in 1958, which was known as the "central dogma of molecular biology." It is essentially a one-way street. This unidirectional pathway of DNA to RNA to proteins essentially means that once information flows to protein, it cannot flow back to RNA or DNA.

However, there are examples where this flow of information is not unidirectional. In "Mad Cow Disease" and in the degenerative brain condition in humans called *Creutzfeldt–Jakob* disease (CJD), scientists thought that any infectious agent that causes these human illnesses had to be in the form of either a DNA or at least a RNA-carrying agent. This dogmatic thinking of DNA to RNA to protein made it hard to identify the infectious agent responsible for this disease. For some time, the possibility that a protein, -- and not a DNA or RNA --could act as an infectious agent was never considered.

In *Creutzfeldt–Jakob* encephalitis and Mad Cow Disease, prions or proteins are the infectious agent. A protein acting as the infectious agent goes against the unidirectional principle of molecular biology. In order for proteins to be an infectious and contagious agent, protein must be "transformed" into DNA or at least RNA. From this example, one can see that the unidirectional pathway of DNA to RNA to protein is indeed false. I believe a bidirectional pathway -- from DNA to RNA to protein or from protein to RNA and DNA-- is possible. A bidirectional pathway from proteins to DNA then makes protein a viable candidate as the material that holds information and memory.

I believe that you can code proteins to RNA and then to DNA. The reason this is possible is that if protein is the "material" that your body uses to store and maintain memory, the protein will need to be stable over time. However, if proteins store data, as do the transistors of a memory chip, protein can break down or become unstable over time. To prevent lapses in memory from the protein being broken down, the protein needs to be in a stable form such as RNA or DNA. In addition, the ability to pass one's life experiences onto the next generation requires passing it via your genetic material -- i.e., DNA.

With this in mind, let's revisit the three forms of cell death. Autophagy-- a self-defense mechanism in dealing with nutritional deficiencies -- is different than necrosis. Necrosis is associated with acute cellular injury from ischemia that then causes the death of the cell. Apoptosis, on the other hand, is an organized cell death since the cell stops dividing by exiting its cell cycle. Apoptosis is a natural process your body uses to maintain its normal organ structure. Without apoptosis the number of cells would be excessive. For instance, if one cell divides to give two cells and these two cells continue to divide to give four cells, you would end up with an abnormal number of cells. If the number of cells that increase through cell division does not equals the same number of cells that dies, an abnormal number of cells would occur. Apoptosis is the body's way of regulating the "perfect" number of cells needs. When the processes of cell division become "unregulated", the cell is able to divide uncontrollably. This cell then becomes a cancer cell— a leading cause of death in our time.

Truth #4

What You Are Eating and Who is Responsible

The issue to consider about nutrition is to understand what you are eating and who is responsible for the nutritional content of the foods you eat daily. The simple answer to this question, is the United States government. The longer answer is the United States government and the food manufacturers. The U.S. government is responsible for the nutritional information that makes up the MY FOOD pyramid system. The governmental agencies assigned to provide specific nutritional information regarding dietary patterns that meet the recommendation for nutritional health are the Department of Health and Human Services (HHS) and the United States Department of Agriculture (USDA). These two agencies are responsible for the Dietary Guidelines for American.

The Dietary Guidelines for Americans (a set of nutrient-based values) was first released in 1980 and revised in 1985, 1990, 1995, 2000, 2005 and most recently December 2010. The Dietary Guidelines for Americans is one form of information used to create the Food Guide Pyramid. The original Food Guide Pyramid developed in 1992 was an educational tool design to help Americans select a healthy diet.

The United States Department of Agriculture uses information from experts of the National Academy of Sciences (NAS) to base their FOOD Guide Pyramid system. President Abraham Lincoln signed into law the National Academy of Sciences on March 3, 1863 as an Act of Congress. The goal of the National Academy of Sciences is to "investigate, examine, experiment, and report upon any subject of science or art" whenever needed by any governmental department. The National Academy of Sciences routinely forms committees to review the latest science regarding nutrition and makes recommendations regarding how you should eat. The U.S. Department of Agriculture can use any nutritional information created by the NAS but is not obligated to do so.

The United States Department of Agriculture is responsible for the Food Guide Pyramid and the Daily Values. (The Daily Values found on food labels provide the consumer with the nutritional information for that food.)

The Food Guide Pyramid

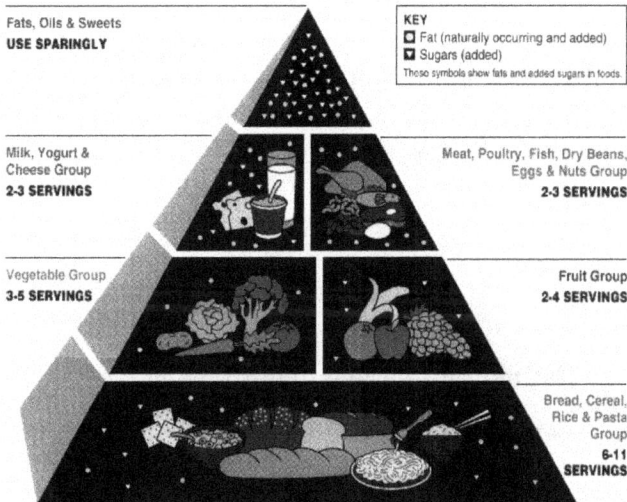

http://en.wikipedia.org/wiki/Food_guide_pyramid

USDA Daily Values for Macronutrients

(Based on a 2000 Calorie Intake)

Nutrient	Unit of Measure	Daily Values (% of daily calories)
Carbohydrate	300 grams	60%
Protein	50 grams	10%
Total Fat	67 grams	30%

The Recommended Dietary Allowances (RDA) is the amount of nutrients believed necessary for your body's daily needs. Today, the RDA is no longer used and was replaced with the Dietary Reference Intakes (DRIs). The DRIs are a combination of information from the Dietary Guidelines for American and the RDA. It is a single recommendation that consumers could use to choose the types and amounts of food to eat daily.

The DRIs for macronutrients published in 2002 includes the following nutrient-based values:

Estimated Average Requirement

Recommended Dietary Allowance (RDA)

Adequate Intake

Tolerable Upper Intake Level

Estimated Energy Requirement

Acceptable Macronutrient Distribution Range (AMDR)

The Dietary Reference Intakes (DRIs) for the macronutrients, expressed as distributive percentages range, is called the Acceptable Macronutrient Distribution Range (AMDR). The current AMDR as recommended by The National Academy of Sciences (NAS) is as follows:

Carbohydrate: 45-65%

Protein: 10-35%

Fat: 20-35%

The AMDR is supposed to provide the essential macronutrients in the amounts needed to reduce the risk for chronic diseases. However, a concern lies in the fact that the AMDR ranges for the macronutrients were used to favor carbohydrate usage. This can be clearly seen within the USDA Daily Values or Food Guide Pyramid. In fact, you will see that it is not balanced since the recommendations overwhelmingly favor carbohydrates over protein.

Depending on the AMDR percentage used, carbohydrate consumption is greater than protein intake by 70% to 600%. Similarly, depending on the percentage range of macronutrients you pick from the NAS AMDR, you could go from a low fat diet pattern, i.e. 60% carbohydrates, 10% proteins, and 30% fats diet pattern, all the way to a "high protein" diet pattern, i.e. Zone diet, in which the percentages of macronutrients are 40% carbohydrates, 30% proteins, 30% fats.

Remember, the key to health and vitality is to eat a diet balanced in the percentage distribution of macronutrients consumed. The Acceptable Macronutrient Distribution Range (AMDR) that represents the Daily Values and the USDA Food

Pyramid system are both reflective of a low fat diet. A low-fat diet-eating pattern is imbalanced in the percentage of carbohydrate to protein to fat and is a highly disguised high carbohydrate diet.

A diet pattern at either extreme, such as a low fat diet or a low carbohydrate diet, is not optimal for health. By recommending more of one macronutrient than another, such as more carbohydrates than protein or fat or more fats than carbohydrate or protein cannot be optimal. The principle of balancing the macronutrients consumed enables optimal health and vitality since individuals who are consuming this type of diet, will likely be in a metabolic state as close to or at homeostasis as possible. In reality, an unbalanced diet pattern, though it can achieve certain goals, is not optimal. It will increase your health risks by stimulating certain homeostatic mechanisms that are acting to control the nutritional imbalances or deficiencies.

Individually, a person's metabolism will dictate which diet patterns will work and which will not. Their current metabolism is determined by their diet over their lifetime. Therefore, the diet pattern that works best for you is not so much genetically determined, but rather nutritionally determined. In truth, no one particular diet pattern will work for every individual, for all situations or at all times. If you agree that a balanced diet pattern is the answer for health, you will be able to learn more as you keep on reading.

As mentioned, the USDA has set the acceptable standard DRI distribution of macronutrients as the Daily Values, which represent the distribution of macronutrients as a percentage of a total daily caloric intake. The Daily Values (DV), are dietary reference values that are supposed to help the consumer use the food label information to plan a healthy diet. The Nutrition Labeling and Education Act of 1990 requires that food labels have information that convey the nutrients found within that food in such a way that the public can observe and comprehend the information and understand its relative significance in context of a total daily diet. The Daily Values is based on a 2,000 calories a day diet.

Example of Nutritional Facts Label

Sample label for
Macaroni & Cheese

① Start Here ➡

② **Check Calories**

③ Limit these Nutrients

④ Get Enough of these Nutrients

⑤ **Footnote**

Nutrition Facts
Serving Size 1 cup (228g)
Servings Per Container 2

Amount Per Serving
Calories 250   Calories from Fat 110

	% Daily Value*
Total Fat 12g	18%
Saturated Fat 3g	15%
Trans Fat 3g	
Cholesterol 30mg	10%
Sodium 470mg	20%
Total Carbohydrate 31g	10%
Dietary Fiber 0g	0%
Sugars 5g	
Protein 5g	

Vitamin A	4%
Vitamin C	2%
Calcium	20%
Iron	4%

*Percent Daily Values are based on a 2,000 calorie diet. Your Daily Values may be higher or lower depending on your calorie needs.

		Calories	2,000	2,500
Total Fat	Less than		65g	80g
Sat Fat	Less than		20g	25g
Cholesterol	Less than		300mg	300mg
Sodium	Less than		2,400mg	2,400mg
Total Carbohydrate			300g	375g
Dietary Fiber			25g	30g

⑥ Quick Guide to % DV

• 5% or less is Low

• 20% or more is High

(Instructions are from the U.S. Food and Drug Administration)

Current Reference Daily Values for the Macronutrients

Daily Values
(Percentage of daily calories based on a 2000 calorie intake)

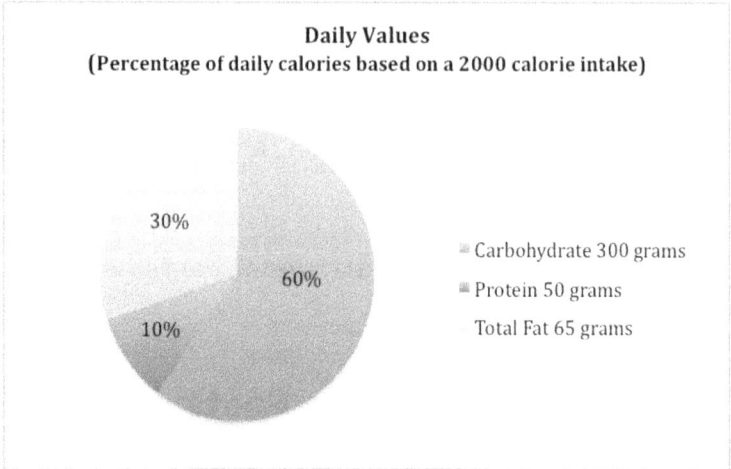

30%

60%

10%

⬛ Carbohydrate 300 grams
⬛ Protein 50 grams
Total Fat 65 grams

Daily Values Calculations Explained

The calculation for the Daily Values is based on a 100 kilogram or 222 pound individual consuming 20 Kcal of calorie per kilogram per day for a total of 2000-calorie daily diet. The reference value for daily fat intake is 65 grams a day, 300 grams of total carbohydrate a day, and 50 grams of protein a day. There are 9 calories per gram of fat so if one consumes 65 grams of fat a day, the calorie contribution in the form of fat in a day is 585 calories. If you did the same for proteins, the calorie contribution is 50 grams per day times 4 calories per gram of protein, or 200 calories per day. A diet with 300 grams of total carbohydrate per day would equal 1200 calories, or 300 grams of carbohydrate times 4 calories per gram of carbohydrate. Dividing 1200 calories of carbohydrate,

200 calories for protein, and 585 calories for fat in a 2000 calorie based diet will give you a 60% carbohydrate, 10% protein, and 30% fat distribution. A 60/10/30 distribution for carbohydrates, proteins, and fats is not a balanced diet in terms of the macronutrients consumed.

One way of determining if an individual is underweight, normal, overweight or obese is to use the body mass index, BMI. The BMI value for a normal weight person is a BMI between 20 and 25. By using a 100-kilogram individual as standard weight for the Daily Values calculation, in order for this 100-kilogram individual to have a BMI less than twenty-five, this individual must be at least six feet and seven inches tall. The majority of individuals I know are not six feet and seven inches. *The actual amount of macronutrients as recommended in the Daily Values is not optimal for health.*

Even though the Daily Values is a low fat diet, it is too high in carbohydrates. The foods that make up a low fat diet pattern are imbalanced in favor of carbohydrates. Remember, a "sugar" is a type of carbohydrate. The term sugar in food labeling is used only for sucrose, table sugar. Starch, a carbohydrate in potatoes, is not considered as a sugar. This comes as a surprise to most of my patients. Many believe that they may be eating too much sugar instead of too much carbohydrate.

A high ratio of any particular macronutrient in a given diet will make that diet imbalanced. Any diet pattern that is imbalanced will not be optimal for health. Looking at the actual grams of carbohydrates within the Daily Values, you will see clearly the inequalities between carbohydrates to that of proteins and fats. A low fat diet pattern has taken the extreme high value for the carbohydrates and low value for the proteins from the NAS recommendations and set them as the standard across all nutritional education.

A quick and useful way to determine the ratio of how much carbohydrate versus protein you are consuming is to look at the food label. The two numbers to focus on within a food label are the total grams of carbohydrate and the total grams of protein. By comparing the ratio of total grams of carbohydrate to the total grams of protein, you will easily see the hidden discrepancy between carbohydrates versus proteins. I will refer to this ratio of total grams of carbohydrate to the total grams of protein as the Carbohydrate to Protein ratio or CP ratio. An optimal nutritional macronutrient CP ratio is one or less. The CP ratio in a low fat diet pattern is at least 6:1 and can be as high as 10:1 or 13:1 of grams of carbohydrate to grams of protein.

It is important to try to understand the goals and motives of the governmental agencies that regulate food nutrition since the guidelines created by them are what food manufacturers use to determine the nutritional value found in the foods you eat daily.

The Wrong-Headed Bias Toward Carbs

By this time, you might be wondering why the current percentages of recommended daily intake for carbohydrates are so high compared to proteins or fats. The reason that the Daily Values is so favorable towards carbohydrate is due to political action taken in 1933.

The truth is that the USDA's involvement and control of what type of foods farmers can grow started during the Great Depression. (The USDA preferences for carbohydrates over proteins and fats increased with president Richard Nixon.) During the Depression, with the stock market crash and falling prices on agriculture commodities, President Franklin D Roosevelt (FDR) created the New Deal programs. Roosevelt's New Deal programs were designed to stimulate the US economy, thereby bringing the Great Depression to an end.

One of the first bills in the New Deal was the creation of the Agriculture Adjustment Act (AAA), enacted on May 12, 1933. The purpose of the AAA, the original Farm Bill, is price control. The AAA was designed to raise crop values by reducing crop surplus. The AAA placed limits on what farmers can grow and cannot grow. It essentially paid farmers to reduce crop production so that crop prices could go higher. The AAA paid farmers to cut production of dairy produce such as milk, butter and livestock.

The money paid to farmers to not farm was made possible through subsidies levied on companies that process farm products. In 1936, the Supreme Court declared the AAA unconstitutional because the money paid to farmers not to farm were taxes levied on the processors. The money generated from food producers was used to pay back the farmers. The Agriculture Adjustment Act of 1938 changed the way in which farmers are now paid. Currently, the money farmers receive to not farm is from general taxation, instead of companies processing farm products.

The reason that the Daily Values are political is that the governmental agency responsible for food nutrition is the USDA. The acronym USDA, of course stands for United States Department of Agriculture. The USDA is responsible for making nutritional recommendations based on scientific information given by the National Academy of Science (NAS).

If you compare the NAS Acceptable Macronutrient Distribution Range with that of the USDA Daily Values, you will see that indeed the USDA followed the NAS recommendations. Why are the gaps in the ranges so great? Since the USDA followed the NAS AMDR recommendations, you would have to wonder why the USDA chose the upper limit for the carbohydrate value at 60% and the lower limit for the protein at 10%?

	ADMR Range	USDA Daily Values
Carbohydrates	45-65%	60%
Proteins	10-35%	10%
Fats	20-35%	30%

By allowing 10% of daily protein intake as an option, the NAS is permitting the USDA to dictate the percentage of macronutrients to use in their favor. The USDA predilection is for agriculture produce foods such as grains and corn versus livestock.

The primary tool the United State Federal Government uses to regulate anything that has to do with agriculture is through the U.S. Farm Bill. The United State Farm Bill is a bill designed for agriculture subsidy. Agriculture subsidy is the way the Federal Government can control prices on such commodities such as wheat, grain feed, cotton, milk, rice, peanuts, sugar, and soybeans. The Federal Government controls commodity prices by regulating what a farmer can or cannot grow. Its ability to control prices on agriculture commodities is one reason for the prevalent use of corn and its derivative product in our foods. Other reasons the US Federal government favors agriculture commodities are 1) the ability to export agriculture commodities to the rest of the world and 2) the desire to find a sustainable food product that can be mass-produced efficiently and at low cost.

To be fair, you can assume that the USDA does not have any hidden agendas and is looking out for your best health interest. Maybe it is their judgment that a higher protein intake is detrimental for your health. If you do research about proteins, what you will find are fears regarding a high protein diet damaging an individual's kidney and liver. There are even reports that a high protein diet might cause osteoporosis and kidney stones. I believe that these fears are just that, fears that are unwarranted because they have been determined false. In fact, recent osteoporosis management recommendations advocate protein intake and do not promote the belief that protein intake causes osteoporosis.

Similarly, at this time there are no upper limits of how much protein a person can take daily that is too much. Protein, when consumed in a balanced amount with other macronutrients and needed micronutrients, is safe and should not be considered harmful. The only possible harm that too much protein intake will cause is greater muscle mass and weight gain due to the conversion of excessive protein to glucose through gluconeogenesis.

Your health is dependent on the micro and macronutrients within the foods you eat. If you recognize which ones are important for health, then you are ahead of most individuals. However, I can speculate that most individuals do not know or possibly care about nutritional guidelines. Most of us just eat foods sold to us in the grocery store by either food recognition, by appearances or taste. In fact, this is how man has survived throughout time, from prehistoric times to the present day. Traditionally, we have eaten foods that are naturally available. However, this is not the case today. Now individuals are eating foods that are genetically modified and supersized by either fertilizer or growth hormones. When you do not understand that the nutrients in foods matter and which foods contain certain nutrients, you just eat foods willy-nilly. Over time you are then at the mercy of the food manufacturers and those that develop the nutritional guidelines. You may trust and believe that the nutritional guidelines we have currently are for your health benefits, but take a second and consider the possibility that that is not true. What would happen if the motives of those that dictate food nutrition or the food manufacturers were not for your health benefit?

Truth #5

Optimal nutrition for Health and Vitality

I began to have a better understanding about nutrition toward the later days of my father's life. This is when I seriously began thinking about ways to improve health. The medical knowledge I had did not help my father as he lay dying. I now know that when I use prescription medications to help my patients with their illnesses or diseases, they do in fact feel better. Yet, for most illnesses or diseases, I never really got a sense that I was doing the most necessary things to slow down or reverse their illnesses or diseases. Moreover, if I did not think of something different than what I already knew, my fate would be the same as my father's. I believe that most of the deaths that occur take place prematurely due to a lack of widespread knowledge regarding nutrition. To improve people's health through nutrition is how I can prevent illnesses and diseases.

Since I have described what optimal nutrition is, I am now going to give examples what it is not. Optimal nutrition is not a solution for all situations. If your goal is to lose weight or gain weight, then optimal nutrition is not the best method to achieve this goal in the quickest amount of time. For weight gain, the amount and distribution of macronutrients that one needs to consume is found in a high calorie, high carbohydrate diet. A diet especially high in calories coming from carbohydrates would give a different result than a diet high in calories derived from fats or proteins.

Let's take the example of two popular diets being promoted today – the Atkins high-fat diet and a low-fat diet – to see how they might affect your overall health goals.

Of the various types of diets out there, each has a different distribution of carbohydrates, proteins, and fats. For example, a low-fat diet is where less than 30% of your calories comes from fat. The fats in this type of diet are often replaced by calories coming from carbohydrates, which will be in the form of grains, fruits and vegetable food groups. The distribution of macronutrients in a low-fat diet is at least 60% carbohydrates, 10% or fewer proteins, and about 30% or less fats in a 60/10/30 distribution. *One of the surprising facts about the food that makes up a low fat diet is that it is mostly carbohydrates!* In fact, it is true that a low fat diet is really a sugar diet, since carbohydrates are sugars.

Diet	Carbohydrate	Protein	Fat
Low Fat	60%	≤ 10%	≤ 30%

However, there are individuals who believe this diet pattern, promoted by the U.S. Department of Agriculture, is incorrect for health and will advocate for the least amount of carbohydrates in the diet such as the Atkins diet. This has caused a battle between the low fat diet advocates verses the low carbohydrate diet pattern advocates. The late Dr. Atkins founded the prototypical low carbohydrate diet pattern for which it is named after him, the Atkins diet. The Atkins diet recommends a 10/20/70 ratio of carbohydrates to proteins to fats.

Diet	Carbohydrate	Protein	Fat
Atkins	10%	20%	70%

The Atkins diet pattern is revolutionary in that it recognizes that eating one type of macronutrient over another offers certain health advantages. For instance, by advocating eating fats instead of carbohydrates as the majority of your calories, the Atkins diet does offer advantages over the low fat diet pattern. However, the Atkins diet pattern suffers from the same criticism as being an imbalanced diet with just a greater intake toward fats. It seems like the Dr. Atkins' diet pattern is essentially a diet pattern that came about as a response to the obesity and health risks from a low fat diet pattern.

A low fat diet pattern tends to cause the overconsumption of carbohydrate calories and thus the person becomes obese from an imbalance in macronutrients consumed. Carbohydrate can be an addictive macronutrient if consumed excessively over time. Ask anyone why they would eat so many carbohydrates and they will say that "they are addicting," and they cannot stop eating them.

A low carbohydrate or the Atkins diet is one that recommends that most of the calories come from fats. An Atkins diet pattern is effective for greater weight loss in a shorter period of time in individuals who are obese to morbidly obese. This diet is the least appetite-stimulating diet pattern since less insulin production is stimulated from the fat consumed. The health benefits of an Atkins diet are different from the low fat diet and are best used when weight loss is desired. However, the Atkins diet's overall health benefits are not as great in individuals of normal weight. In addition, the amount of protein recommended in a traditional Atkins diet, 20% of total calories consumed, is lower then those I believe needed for optimal health, which is at least 35%.

Conversely, a low fat diet pattern will result in increased appetite and obesity over time. Composing of mostly carbohydrates, a low fat diet stimulates insulin release, fat deposition, and increase appetite. It's also the reason why grain and corn feeds are used to fatten livestock in the shortest time that's possibly needed for market.

The USDA Daily Values for an individual weighing 100 kilograms is 300 grams per day of carbohydrates, 50 grams per day of proteins, and 65 grams per day of fats. The diet pattern advocated for health by the USDA is a low fat diet pattern. This is evident from the My Food Pyramid and the Acceptable Macronutrient Distribution Range (AMDR) of the Daily Values. These AMDR values are too low in proteins and too high in carbohydrates for optimal long-term health. We need to re-examine the AMDR if we want to find the answers to health and vitality.

The distribution of the macronutrients for both the low fat and low carbohydrate diet such as an Atkins diet can vary in the macronutrient distribution but for all purposes, the percentages I have given is close enough for discussion. The low fat diet and the Atkins diet pattern are both diets that work for different purposes and for different individuals.

For individuals who want to lose weight effectively, the diet pattern best suited for this purpose is a low carbohydrate diet pattern such as the Atkins diet. An Atkins diet pattern focuses most of the macronutrient calories in the form of fats (70%) and has the least amount of carbohydrate calories (10%). Eating an Atkins diet pattern will lessen the chance for weight gain, due to the lower insulin level, unlike a low fat diet that offers a greater chance for weight gain. For some followers of the Atkins diet pattern, there exists an incorrect assumption that a food calorie does not matter in the mechanism of obesity. Simply stated, they believe that it is simply the overconsumption of carbohydrate that causes weight gain and obesity and that the total calories consumed do not matter if they happen to be fat.

A major factor contributing to the obesity epidemic is the overconsumption of carbohydrates. Yet, believing that it is carbohydrates only and that the total amount of calories consumed does not play a role in weight gain or loss is incorrect. Food calories do matter in determining a person's weight. How much food calories eaten per day do matter toward your weight. This is true even if those food calories happen to be fat. Atkins supporters believe that calories do not matter in the dynamic process of weight gain or loss. The reason the Atkins eating pattern works for weight loss is that it eliminates most carbohydrates from your diet and replaces it with fats. Eliminating the overconsumption of carbohydrates will negate the normal metabolic processes that tend to promote weight gain, which is fat deposition.

An Atkins eating pattern is less detrimental to your health than a low fat eating pattern regarding its effect on weight gain. Yet for issues such as long-term health effects, an Atkins eating pattern is not optimal for health. The reason for this is that an Atkins diet is still too extreme a pattern, which focuses mostly on fats. Fats for health are okay, but not in the extremes seen in an Atkins diet pattern. Imbalances of macronutrients in any dietary eating pattern, whether it is in carbohydrates, proteins or fats, is not optimal. Had Dr. Atkins stressed the importance of a greater dietary intake of proteins along with fats, his diet plan would have had a greater acceptance and would be a true revolution in health. A diet balanced with carbohydrates, proteins, and fats would win more people over.

Consumption of fats has less weight gain potential since its metabolism is different then carbohydrates. However, the emphasis on fats in this diet is not optimal nutrition since the macronutrients are still imbalanced. From this discussion, you can see that the dietary pattern of a low fat diet pattern versus the Atkins diet -- each achieves certain goals yet have opposing health effects.

Weight loss occurs by one of two ways, by increasing metabolism and keeping caloric intake the same, or by taking in fewer calories than what your body is accustomed to, essentially causing a calorie deficit. Generally, you can lose one pound of body weight when there is a deficit of thirty-five hundred calories. For example, if you eat five hundred calories less each day, over a week's time, you should in theory lose one pound of body weight.

A Calorie Is Just a Calorie...Or Is It?

I have just brought calories into the discussion of nutrition. Food calories and their effect on your weight and health should be a straightforward issue. The simple fact is that the more calories you consume, the greater your weight will be over time. Yet, the effects of these calories on your weight are currently a topic of hot debate. Some believe that carbohydrate consumption causes weight gain, while fat consumption does not. I am about to disprove this assumption. I will shed light on the topic of food calories by explaining some misassumptions about the lowly calorie. The widely held view about a food calorie is that a "calorie is a calorie," when it comes to gaining weight or losing weight. What this principle means for weight loss or gain is "calories in, calories out." Individuals who believe in the "calories in, calories out" principle think weight gain or loss is due the amount of food calories eaten. Thus, obesity is a disorder of too many calories in. Conversely, weight loss is possible when you eat fewer calories.

Calculating the Calories You Would Need to Remain at Your Current Weight (low physical activity)

Weight(lbs) X 10 kcal(food calorie) = Daily Caloric Requirement

---

Another concept tied to the "calorie is a calorie," equation is that carbohydrate and protein both contain approximately 4 kcal of energy per gram of food. Fat is different since it possesses approximately double the amount of calories of carbohydrate or protein. Fat has 9 kcal per gram of potential energy. Up to this point, everything said about a food calorie is a fact. Why "a calorie is a calorie" and the "calories in, calories out" concept are both true is that the metabolism of macronutrients is different than the energy potential that these foods possess. The assumption is that the metabolism of a carbohydrate, protein, and fat has to be the same because they each have food calorie qualites. This is a false assumption. The metabolism of a carbohydrate is different than a protein or that of a fat.

The reason Atkins supporters refuse to accept the concept of a "calories in, calories out," is that they know that fat metabolism is different than that of carbohydrates. Individuals who advocate the Atkins diet do so because fat does not cause as much weight gain compared to a diet based on carbohydrates. The fact that your body metabolizes fat differently than a protein or a carbohydrate is not hard to understand. Carbohydrates stimulate insulin release. High insulin from high carbohydrate consumption promotes fat deposition. Protein and fat do not stimulate insulin release the same way and thus do not promote the fat deposits seen with carbohydrates.

The reason why "a calorie is a calorie," and the "calories in, calories out" principle is disputed by Atkins supporters is that they are forgetting what a food calorie represents. Let's harken back to our high school physics: A calorie represents a unit of energy. Professor Nicolas Clement first defined a calorie in 1824 as a unit of heat -- a calorie was the unit of energy required to raise the temperature of one gram of water by 1 °C. Since a calorie is a measurement of energy, the concept that one calorie equals another calorie is true. What the concept of "a calorie is a calorie," does not state is that a macronutrient possessing one food calorie is metabolized the same as another macronutrient possessing one food calorie.

Translated, a carbohydrate, protein, and fat are not metabolized the same way. Only the energy potential that each macronutrient possesses in calories per gram is comparable. Therefore, eating an excessive amount of calories in the form of carbohydrates will contribute more weight gain than calories from proteins or fats.

Everything in Moderation

When you think about nutrition, forget what you have learned about the food pyramid. Do not think about nutrition so much in terms of what certain foods look like or taste like. How a food looks or tastes is important. Yet, realizing that how a food looks or tastes is often artificial and may make one choosier. *Learn to think about foods in terms of the nutrients within them and you will understand why over eating certain foods can lead to nutritional imbalances.*

Like the saying "a rose by any other name," a sugar is a carbohydrate and vice versa. Eating too much of one macronutrient over another is the cause for many of the illnesses and diseases we have today. Some people believe fructose, a type of carbohydrate in the form of high fructose corn syrup (HFCS), causes obesity and certain diseases. It is true that too much fructose can have adverse health affects. However, remember, fructose is still a carbohydrate and is not necessarily bad when consumed in moderation. It is the overconsumption of fructose that is causing the problems and not fructose itself.

This gives me a chance to reiterate an important point about optimal health and nutrition: It is about a balanced diet pattern of needed micronutrients and macronutrients. Overconsumption of any macronutrient is not a good idea.

I will outline the ideal percentage of macronutrients needed in an optimal diet pattern for health. Key points to think about any diet:

1) Consider the distribution of macronutrients needed versus those found in your diet

2) Provide enough of those needed micro and macronutrients daily

Knowing and fulfilling these two factors will enable you to function optimally since your body will be metabolically in equilibrium (homeostasis).

Let's examine what most individuals are eating. Most of us are eating foods that come from the typical grocery store. They arrive in the house either as raw ingredients such a fresh fruits, vegetables, and raw meats or they are in the form of pre-packaged processed foods that are ready for you to eat (pre-packaged, frozen or canned).

By eating pre-packaged processed foods, the outcome of your long-term health is determined by the food manufacturers. When food manufacturers follow the USDA Daily Values nutritional profile, chances are you are eating at least 60% carbohydrates, less than 30% fats, and definitely less then the 35% protein recommended as the high range for daily protein intake by the National Academy of Science (NAS) Acceptable Macronutrient Distribution Range (AMDR). The actual amount of protein that you are getting from most pre-packaged foods is probably about 10% or less of the total daily caloric intake.

The total amount of daily protein you need should be dependent on your body weight. The more you weigh the more protein you need. Currently, your body weight is not a factor in the actual calculation of the amount of proteins needed daily.

A daily protein intake of 10% of total caloric intake is about 0.25 gram of protein per pound of body weight. For an individual weighing one hundred pounds, 10% protein intake of total calories is 25 grams of protein a day. In physical food form, 25 grams of protein is a little bit over three ounce of meat such as red meat, pork, chicken or fish. A three-ounce serving of food is about the size of a deck of playing cards. One ounce of meat has about 7 grams of protein. A deck of card serving size has 21 grams of protein. Consuming 10% of your total caloric intake as protein is insufficient for your daily needs. This amount will cause protein malnutrition over time.

The reasons for protein deficiency are many and complex. One reason is that the USDA Daily Values for the macronutrients is imbalanced. This point is important since the USDA sets the nutritional guideline that food manufacturers have to follow in the type of foods to produce. Therefore, if the USDA food pyramid system and Daily Values are incorrect, then food manufacturers can produce foods that contain an imbalance of the needed macronutrients. Currently, the nutritional information from the USDA food pyramid system and Daily Values are taken as standards for everyone to follow.

Another reason for protein deficiency is due to the dietary eating patterns that individuals are following. The standard dietary recommendation for an individual with cardiovascular disease or high cholesterol is a low fat diet pattern. This is to be accomplished by avoiding fats within their diet by not eating red meat. I believe this recommendation has unintended consequences for your health. *Avoiding red meat or meat in general due to fats will increase the chances that your protein intake will worsen over time.* The truth is that you can still eat red meats -- in moderation.

In fact, as long as the fat content is not excessively high, with no more than 35% fat content, then eating almost any type of food is okay. In addition, a recommendation to avoid red meat as a way to lower your blood lipids fails to address the true reason why high blood cholesterol is occurring. The cause for high blood cholesterol (hypercholesterolemia) in most individuals is not so much due to eating fats as it is due to eating too many foods that are carbohydrates. A diet deficient in red meats (a good source of proteins) will likely exacerbate protein malnutrition over an extended period.

The reason why avoiding red meat is worrisome advice is that most individuals' diet pattern is already inherently low in protein intake needed for their body weight. Avoiding red meat will just magnify the severity of protein deficiency in individuals who follow this advice. The advice to avoid fats and cholesterol-rich foods as a way to lower your cholesterol is misguided. The reason for this is that dietary fat intake is not the real reason for your high blood cholesterol.

Eating a low fat diet will cause high blood cholesterol since this diet pattern is full of carbohydrate-rich foods. A diet full of carbohydrate rich foods will stimulate your liver to begin endogenous cholesterol biosynthesis. The mechanism behind high blood cholesterol, as we've discussed, is due to endogenous cholesterol synthesis by your liver and not from eating fats found in meats. Dietary intestinal cholesterol absorption is minimal compared to the actual amount of cholesterol synthesis by your liver when you consume too many carbohydrates.

Avoiding saturated fats is not necessarily good nutritional advice. Eating saturated fats in moderation is beneficial, since this is where the fat-soluble vitamins are stored. This point of not getting enough fat-soluble vitamins through eating fats is not recognized. When one tries to avoid foods that contain fats, the likelihood of proteins and fat-soluble vitamins deficiencies are greater. Other sources of foods that have protein and essential fatty acid are foods such as soybean and nuts. However, these foods will not have the same quantity of protein as that found from animal sources. If you eat a vegetarian diet, please be sure that you choose a combination of protein sources that has all the essential amino acids and some of the vitamins and minerals not readily found in a vegetarian diet.

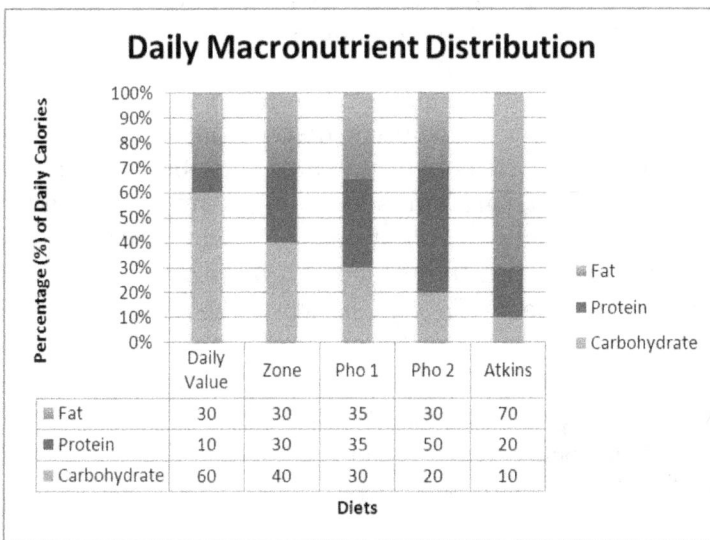

Daily Macronutrient Distribution

	Daily Value	Zone	Pho 1	Pho 2	Atkins
Fat	30	30	35	30	70
Protein	10	30	35	50	20
Carbohydrate	60	40	30	20	10

Diets

The ideal distribution for the macronutrients needed for health is 30% carbohydrates or less, at least 35%-40% proteins, and about 30% lipids. I believe that the distribution of macronutrients needed in terms of carbohydrates, proteins, and fats (CPF) is somewhere between a 30/35/35 (CPF) to a potential 20/50/30 (CPF) distribution. From this discussion, you can see that the dietary pattern of a low fat diet pattern versus the Atkins diet -- each achieves certain goals yet have opposing health effects.

A 30/35/35 percentage distribution of carbohydrates, to proteins, to lipids ratio is more of a balanced ratio than the current 60/10/30 percentage distribution of the Daily Values recommendation. A 40/30/30 diet pattern is a pattern characteristic of The Zone diet. However, the distribution of macronutrients I advocate differs from The Zone diet in that the protein percentage is at least 35%, while the carbohydrate percentage should be less than or equal to 30%.

A higher percentage distribution of protein is favored over carbohydrate and fat because as a macronutrient, protein serves a greater importance than carbohydrates or fats. Protein serves as a function beyond a fuel source; it plays a vital function in every aspect of your health. The percentage of protein needed for health, at least 35%, does not make it a high protein diet. It is considered high only when your standard is at the low end -- 10%. (Refer to the reference section of the book for calculations about different type of diets.)

Avoiding a Protein Deficiency

Deficiencies or over-abundances of food nutrients can happen to anyone of us. It happened to my father, and it even happened to me. The information regarding nutrition that you need to understand is that the current body of information regarding nutrition is confusing, impractical, and not followed. *The current recognized medical recommendation for the Recommended Dietary Allowance (RDA) for proteins in the United States, for an adult is 0.8 grams per kilogram per day.* This standard for daily protein intake was set in 1974.

This 0.8 grams per kilogram of protein per day is equivalent to about 0.37 gram of protein per pound of body weight per day. Therefore, for an individual weighing one hundred pounds, the total amount of protein needed would be 37 grams of protein. These 37 grams of protein represent 15% of the total daily calories consumed for an individual weighing one hundred pounds who is using about 10 kcal of energy per pound per day (for an inactive person).

Medically, a baseline of at least 0.8 gram per kilogram or 0.37 gram per pound of body weight for protein is required daily. The current protein intake from the USDA Daily Values is not based on 0.8 grams per kilogram of protein intake or a 15% of the total daily calories but at a lower percentage of 10% of total caloric intake. This 10% of total caloric intake is about fifty grams of protein a day in a standard 2000 kcal (food calorie) per day diet. The USDA Daily Value protein intake of 10% is lower than the RDA minimal 15% of the total daily caloric intake. This discrepancy should alert you of trouble coming. The USDA Daily Value for daily protein intake needs to be increased to at least the minimal 15% of total calories and not be at the low 10%.

Optimally, the amount of proteins needed daily could really be about 2 grams per kilogram or 1 gram per pound of body weight. The increase is needed because it will then give you 40% of your daily caloric intake as protein instead of the 10% of daily caloric intake as it currently stands. The 2 grams per kilogram or 1 gram per pound of body weight for proteins would then represent a 400% increase from the current USDA Daily Value baseline of 10% of total calories.

The information you need to know is the amount of protein needed daily for proper health. By knowing this, you can then figure out for yourself if you are actually eating enough protein daily. The actual amount of protein that any of us consumes daily is variable due to our choices of foods to eat. However, as stated before, the food manufacturers, along with regulatory agencies such as the USDA, will determine in some part how much protein you will consume simply due to the amount of protein they allow for nutritional health. The amount of protein that is considered adequate for health is currently dictated by the USDA Daily Value at 10% of total caloric intake or about fifty grams of protein a day for a standard 2000 kcal per day diet. For those of you who are just getting this 10% of total caloric intake or about fifty grams of protein a day requirement, be careful -- you likely have protein malnutrition.

If you are not meeting the USDA Daily Value protein requirement of 10% of total caloric intake or about fifty grams of protein a day, you have a lot of catching up to do. Consider that it is not even the minimal amount needed for health. How the 10% of total caloric intake of protein amount came about will be discussed later.

The minimal daily amount of protein medically recommended is 0.8 gram per kilogram of body weight or 15% of your total daily caloric intake. The 0.8 gram per kilogram per day of protein intake is the minimal amount needed daily to maintain lean body muscle mass. For general purposes, even the 0.8 gram per kilogram per day of daily-required protein intake, is in my opinion, still inadequate.

The actual amount of protein you need daily for optimal health is probably 2 grams per kilogram per day, or one gram per pound daily. For a one hundred pound individual, this amount is approximately one hundred grams of protein daily or the equivalent of fourteen ounces of meat or about five serving of meat a day. You might think that this amount of protein is too much and is impossible given the way you are eating now. You are right about not being able to get enough protein needed for your body weight if you continue to eat those foods you are eating now. However, you are incorrect to say this amount of protein is too much. For example, toddlers who drink 4 to 5 cups of milk a day are probably getting about a gram of protein per pound daily. The issue is that you cannot continue to eat the same way you are currently eating. You will have to change by eating fewer cereals, grains, fruits, vegetables and carbohydrate based foods. You will need to eat more protein-based foods such as meats. Eating protein-based foods was what people did in the early 1900's and definitely before the advent of industrial farming.

The reasons no one is going to tell you how much protein you actually need daily is because of two possible explanations. The first and most logical is that "we" just do not yet understand the importance of protein in health. The second answer is not a pleasant answer and not as "politically correct" as the first. The reason protein based foods are not emphasized is that those that should "know better" are either are too busy trying to support a cause or have a motive that is politically or monetarily based. The production and promotion of agricultural food products that are profitable and yet harmful for health, prevent the truth from coming out.

The recommended amount of daily protein intake for anyone younger than an adult is even higher. The National Academy of Science (NAS) RDA recommendation for daily protein for infants is 1.5 grams per kilogram per day. For those 1 to 3 years old, the RDA for protein intake is 1.1 grams per kilogram per day. For the 4 to 13 years old, the RDA for protein intake is 0.95 grams per kilogram per day. For those 14-18 years old, the RDA for protein intake is 0.85 grams per kilogram per day.

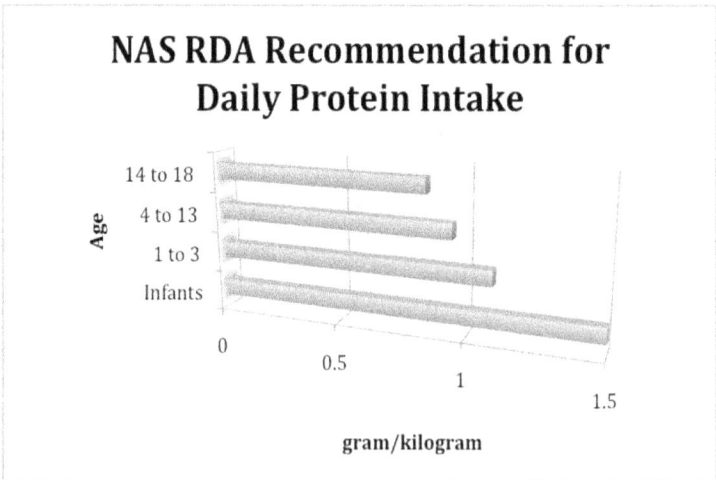

NAS RDA Recommendation for Daily Protein Intake

Age: 14 to 18, 4 to 13, 1 to 3, Infants

gram/kilogram (0, 0.5, 1, 1.5)

In looking at the above NAS RDA for protein intake, one can see that the recommended daily protein intake decreases as you age. The evidence and logic in support of decreasing one's daily protein intake as you age is questionable. Nevertheless, the current belief is that you require less daily protein intake as you age.

Let's examine this argument: Nutrition is one factor that determines your health. The other factor contributing to your health is genetics. Genetic inheritance or susceptibility you cannot change. For instance, you cannot change your hair or skin color. However, compared to nutrition, genetics has more of a secondary role in your overall health than you realize. After you are born, nutrition, and environmental factors, determine what genetic feature is expressed. You can think of genetics as the blueprint. Yet, nutrition is the main factor that affects how the blueprint is played out.

The fate of over consuming proteins is similar to carbohydrates. Protein consumed in excessive amounts will not be stored as protein. The excess will be stored as fats but ONLY after your body uses the needed amino acids. You therefore do not have any stored forms of protein in your body, except possibly your muscles. Every amino acid within a protein that you consume and possess is serving a purpose within your body. Examples of protein currently performing vital functions in your body are enzymes, muscles, and connective tissues found in your body.

The tissues beneath the surface of your skin are connective tissues and are made of protein. These connective tissues are what keep you looking young. As you "age," the elasticity of your skin is lost. The reason this happens is that your skin has lost the supportive structure provided by the connective tissues beneath your skin. The reason given why you lose the supportive structure provided by your connective tissues, as you get older, is that of aging. However, a better explanation as to why you are losing the supportive connective tissues' structure is due to a protein and subcutaneous fat deficiency exacerbated over your lifetime. Protein deficiencies happen daily and over time result in the loss of elasticity of your skin from the loss of connective tissues. Recognizing the possibility that protein malnutrition presents as skin wrinkles will help you realize that protein deficiency could cause your health to deteriorate in other ways.

Dietary proteins consumed are broken down in your small intestine by enzymes called peptidase into individual amino acids. The likelihood that the needed quantities of the individual or essential amino acids are available depends on the food source eaten. Once the amino acids are absorbed into your bloodstream, it is used for the synthesis of needed structural proteins, enzymes or even as a backup source of fuel. Any free amino acids in your bloodstream will be used and is not "stored" as free amino acids. Every amino acid in your bloodstream will eventually be used. Certain amino acids are able to undergo gluconeogenesis to glucose when the glucose level becomes low, such as a high metabolic state. Consuming more amino acids than needed will cause them to undergo transformation into glucose and then fats if the transformed glucose is not used immediately.

From the discussion above, you can now see how nutritional deficiencies can develop. They may develop slowly and insidiously in the background of daily life. Nutritional deficiencies can develop at any time when your body is not getting an adequate amount of proteins, fats, vitamins and minerals daily.

Because of this, the root causes of human illnesses and diseases are linked to nutritional deficiencies.

During the repair, replacement and maintenance processes of your cells, your body will recycle most of the nutrients from the cells that were replaced. *The recycling of nutrients from "dying" cells decreases the actual amount of new nutrients needed.* This recycling process reduces the possibility of subtle nutritional deficiencies that would otherwise occur. Recycling is an inherent process available to our body that buys us time so that we can replenish nutritional deficiencies. However, having said this, what happens if the deficient nutrients continue to be deficient? You have a tipping point for illnesses or disease. There can be single or multiple events that contribute to the tipping point. If you want to avoid such events, then adequate nutrition is required daily. I believe if the needed micro and macronutrients are optimal; your body would not need to recycle as many nutrients as it does in a nutritionally deficient state. To use recycle nutrients or have new nutrients? You decide.

The reason why nutritional deficiencies are not readily apparent is due to the process called autophagy. Autophagy, or really, the recycling of nutrients, is one of the three processes in which a cell can die. As you probably remember, cell death occurs by necrosis, apoptosis and autophagy. Autophagy is a process in which the body wills itself out of necessity to "eat" itself for the needed nutrients. Your body does this even if the cell parts that are "eaten" are not "broken" and are serving essential functions. *If the micro and macronutrients needed from your diet are not available, then your body will use autophagy as a way to seize the resources it needs.*

The explanation given as to why older individuals lose muscle mass is aging. The medical term for the loss of muscle mass related to age is sarcopenia. However, aging is often the explanation given to those processes that occur, as you get older and have no explanation for its etiology. There are logical explanations, besides aging, for the loss of muscle mass seen in the elderly. Ask the question of why a person should lose muscle mass to an athlete or a body builder, and chances are they can tell you the correct answer. Here is a hint: do not consider the age of an individual and just ask yourself what causes a person to lose lean muscle mass. The athlete and body builder will not say that aging is the reason a person loses muscle mass. Their answer as to why muscle mass is lost would be due to the lack of adequate proteins needed to maintain it.

The inability to sustain an adequate daily protein intake required for body weight is the reason muscle mass is lost. This fact is true regardless of age. Whether you are young or old, muscle mass is sacrificed once adequate sources of proteins are not there to supply the amino acids needed. Inadequate protein intake will cause your body to start breaking down the lean muscle mass by the process of autophagy. When dietary proteins are unmet due to deficiencies or increased demand, muscle mass is lost. This example is just the tip of a larger problem stemming from a deficiency of protein that occurs over time.

I have discussed the importance of nutrition on health in the sense of giving our body the optimal amount of nutrients needed. At this time, I do not believe that we actually know the optimal amount needed for each of the micronutrients and macronutrients. This information needs to be determined so that we can achieve optimal health.

For those of you who are not getting either the fifty grams of protein a day or the 0.8 gram per kilogram of protein daily, reconsider if you think a higher daily protein intake recommendation is something you would like to follow. Another point that you need to consider is to look at the source of proteins you are consuming. The type of foods that you eat can be significant in the sense of the available quantity and quality of proteins found in the food. This point is important for those who are vegetarians. For those that are vegetarians, what you need to know, is the source of proteins you are eating needs to be complete, with both the essential and nonessential amino acids. Cereal, corn, or grain-based foods are incomplete proteins since they lack the essential amino acid lysine.

Eat Local; Eat Whole Foods

The holy grail of health and vitality is when your body is in or at homeostasis. The reason why any diet patterns or supplements work to improve your health is if it leads your body toward homeostasis. Any diet patterns that work, work because they enable you to be closer to homeostasis than the one you were previously eating. Enabling an ever-closer state of homeostasis to improve health explains why such things as any medications, foods, herbs, supplements, physical activities or religion also work to enhance it. For example, the reason that eating fresh, local whole foods is beneficial is that your body is getting more of the nutrients it needs to be in homeostasis without having to deal with deficiencies of nutrients or toxins and chemicals from the food itself. This is the principle of "organic" foods.

Let us discuss in depth why eating fresh, local whole foods are beneficial for you. Foods such as fruits and vegetables available out of season are convenient, but these conveniences come at a cost to your health. By eating fresh foods, you are not at the mercy of the USDA Daily Values or food manufacturers and any possible negative health effects from processed foods will not be an issue. By eating "locally grown" foods, you decrease the chances of having foods that have been treated with chemicals to ripen or to maintain the "shelf" life of the foods you are eating. Eating whole foods is beneficial because they have a greater amount of nutrients than eating refined processed foods. For those that are environmentally conscious, eating local grown foods will also decrease the carbon "footprint" of manufactured foods' effect on the environment.

When you are thinking about organic foods, you are trying to improve health by providing your body with natural nutrients. The health benefits of eating organic foods are that they have fewer chemicals and pesticides use in their growth, processing and final product for your consumption. It is true that eating foods with fewer nutrients and more chemicals or toxins can adversely affect your health.

To make sense of what the organic versus processed foods argument really means, think of it this way: Processed foods are for your convenience and the desire for speed of having it "all right here and now." You want the food to be affordable, fast and good tasting. You have asked for it, and the food industries have complied. Processed foods will not only have fewer micronutrients, they are also loaded with that all too familiar macronutrient, carbohydrates. Similarly, processed foods will have chemicals not naturally found in nature. These effects will likely causes imbalances of needed micro and macronutrients to occur over time. As for organic foods, the opposite of what I have said about processed foods applies.

Use Supplements Wisely

How do we now fix those problems I have raised? The answer is to realistically look at nutrition and find a solution that you can follow. From the health effects of processed foods versus organic foods, it cannot be assumed that organic foods are the answer to improve your health. Organic food provides the "purer" form of micro and macronutrients needed but not necessarily in the correct percentages needed. Only knowledge in selecting the right food micro and macronutrients will provide the correct amount needed. As a long-term solution, foods that provide the needed micro and macronutrients in the amount required for health are ideal. Deficient micro and macronutrients adversely affect your health and are harder to make up over time. In addition, no one food exists, whether it is organic or not, has all the micro and macronutrients needed in the optimal amount.

This opens the door for supplements. The benefit of supplementation is that you can systematically use any micro and macronutrients to correct nutritional deficiencies from the foods you eat daily. A given food may have the micro and macronutrients needed but lack the quantity needed. Alternatively, the amount of micronutrients from fruits you would need is hard to obtain without getting too much of certain other macronutrients, such as carbohydrates. So what nutrients should you supplement? You should supplement any nutrients that are likely to be deficient or eaten in inadequate amounts. This requires that you put in some effort in order to know what type of foods you are eating and what nutrients to supplement. The nutrients needing supplementation, due to most individual health status and eating habits are proteins, vitamins, minerals, and the essential fatty acids.

A Review of How Much Protein to Consume

The amount of protein needed daily is specific to your body weight. The minimal amount of protein needed in grams per day is at least half your body weight in pounds. For individuals weighting one hundred pounds, this is equal to fifty grams of protein a day. The amount of protein that is half your body weight in pounds is equal to 20% of your total caloric intake. If you increase your total caloric intake from twenty to either possibly 40-50%, the amount of proteins needed is now equal to one gram to 1.25 grams per pound of body weight daily. I do not make a recommendation for carbohydrate intake, not because it is unimportant, but because most individuals normally consume enough carbohydrates daily. (See the appendix at the end of book for the calculation.)

Take a second to consider the difference between the current amounts of protein recommended per day for a normal adult, 10% of total daily caloric intake, and what a 40-50% of total daily caloric intake really mean for your health. This amount is at least four times greater than that recommended from the current Daily Values. At first glance, you might think this amount is too high and impossible to consume as a food source. Believe me, not only is up to 40% of your total daily caloric intake needed, it is used by athletes and is the minimal amount of protein consume by body builders. Body builders and weight lifters are consuming a minimal of one gram to a high of 2 grams of protein per pound of body weight daily. You might wonder why there is such a wide gap in what body builders and weight lifters are consuming versus the

Daily Values. This difference makes you wonder which recommendations to believe. A body builder can consume anywhere from one to two grams of protein per pound per day while the current Daily Values for an adult is only 0.25 grams of protein per pound per day or 10% of total caloric intake.

The reasons for the differences in the current Daily Values and that of the body builder are many. One reason is that the Daily Value protein recommendation represents just the bare minimal amount of protein needed and not the optimal or maximal amount of protein needed daily. Remember, the AMDR daily protein intake ranges are 10-35% of daily caloric intake. By setting the Daily Value for protein intake at 10%, the USDA has guided nutrition education to believe this as the standard "optimal" amount. Not surprisingly, another problem with the Daily Values is the daily carbohydrate intake is set at 60% of total daily calories. This value is close to the upper limit of carbohydrate intake recommended by the NAS Acceptable Macronutrient Distribution Range (AMDR) recommendation.

Truth #6

The Straw That Broke the Camel's Back

The saying goes that "a picture can speak a thousand words." Therefore, when I say, "The Straw That Broke the Camel's back," can you imagine a straw actually breaking a camel's back? Of course, that cannot actually happen, you say. And yes, you are right. The truth is that this is just a figurative saying meaning that so much was piled on the camel's back that he couldn't take anything else. What this something else can be is the question. For health, this something else is an event or set of events that when set in motion, will break the camel's back.

Another way of thinking about what broke the camel's back, the final act, is what I will refer to as the "tipping point." The first time I heard this phrase "The Tipping Point," is from Malcolm Gladwell book, "*The Tipping Point*." For those that have read this book, you are familiar with this terminology and its implied meaning. For those that have not, an example of a tipping point event concerning your health is as follows: It is the point at which the delicate balance between your usual normal states of health shifts to a different and changed state. This shift is usually from good health to illness and disease. Rarely, the shift is opposite, from ill health to good health.

Your predisposition for health or illness is determined by both internal and external factors. The internal factor that affects your health is your genetic makeup. The external factor that affects your health is your environment. The environmental factor that has the greatest impact on your health is your nutrition, or, simply put, the foods you eat daily. These will keep you alive and if the nutrients within them are adequate, possibly healthy. Other factors that act on your health are your daily activity level and stressors. These stressors are the metabolic demands on your nutritional reservoir. They can lead to a tipping point event when your metabolic demand depletes your limited nutritional reservoir. This final act or tipping point will result in a significant health change.

One way to illustrate this concept is that of the low gasoline warning indicator meter or light found in cars. Once the light for the low gasoline indicator turns on, you have a limited time before the car will no longer operate. Now think of the car's low gasoline indicator in the same way as your sensation of hunger and thirst. When you get hungry or thirsty, you will satisfy these sensations by eating or drinking. Hunger and thirst are comparable to the car's low gasoline indicator. If you do not eat and drink or fill the gasoline tank when the car's low gasoline light comes on, your body or the car will eventually cease to function.

The take away point about hunger, thirst, or the car's low gasoline indicator is that it is an indicator for an impending deficiency in fuel needed to run "the engine." Your survival -- or the functional operation of the car -- will stop if hunger or the low gasoline light indicator is not addressed. The critical point about hunger, thirst, or a car's low gasoline indicator is that they only warn you of the need to supply fuel for your body or gasoline for the car. They do not warn you of any other potential deficiencies of other nutrients needed for health.

You do not have a warning indicator for any potential deficiencies of any specific micro or macronutrients. The only indicator your body has is for the need to eat foods for food calories. Eating foods without realizing the imbalances of the micro and macronutrients found within them will adversely affect your health. Any food calories you eat will keep you alive just by filling your body's gas tank, which is your stomach. Eating food lacking the nutrients needed to keep you healthy will cause you to break down over time. You can take care of your body by providing it with the needed micro and macronutrients that will keep you healthy.

Real life examples of tipping point events I often hear from my patients are to describe their health as, "I was healthy or fine until I turned ----." A similar statement is, "I was healthy or fine until this X event happened to me." The age or the X event can be any age or events you wish to make it. The point is that some individuals often describe their health as being fine at one point in time and worse the next point in time. What are the explanations or reasons for this type of events? Can a person's health really deteriorate because of any single event or age? Can your health swing in the balance from being good at one moment to being ill and sick simply because you are one year older? Can any event really change your health for the worse? After hearing these types of comments, I began to think about how to explain these events. I wanted to find out how your health can indeed change from one moment to the next.

The straw that broke the camel's back or the tipping point represents a point in time where things just seem to happen that did not happen before. In health, the straw and the tipping point are points in time where nutritional deficiencies that developed slowly throughout your lifetime become relevant and significant enough to finally affect your health. Once a nutritional deficiency occurs, the likelihood is that it will continue and worsen over time. Nutritional deficiencies do not happen overnight and often occur slowly, over time. They also tend to worsen because you do not have a "warning" gauge for any nutrients you are missing. By continuing your habits of eating certain not-so-healthy foods, your body and health will slowly deteriorate over time.

I have described hunger, thirst and a car's low gasoline indicator as an indicator for the need to fuel "our engine." A point to consider next is, since you do not have any other indicators or warning light, how will you know if you are deficient in a certain nutrient? The answer is, you will not. You will never know since there is no warning indicator for any nutrients beside hunger as the need to eat and thirst as the need to drink.

Individuals with nutritional deficiencies will present with signs and symptoms of illnesses that will be diagnosed as a medical condition. But treating signs and symptoms or medical diagnoses will not improve your health. This is different than addressing nutritional deficiencies. Addressing nutritional deficiencies is the first step to treating root causes for illnesses and diseases. Illnesses and diseases do not arise in a vacuum. Illnesses and diseases are causally linked to deficient nutrients. The recognition and acceptance of this principle will be the first step in addressing the root causes for illnesses and diseases.

An example of a nutritional deficiency that develops over time is that of vitamin D. Vitamin D is an important hormone needed for calcium regulation. Over time, due to the lack of ultraviolet B radiation exposure, you can become vitamin D deficient. The lack of vitamin D will not have any noticeable ill effects unless you recognize the signs and symptoms of vitamin D deficiency. Similarly, protein deficiency is now very common. Protein deficiencies are occurring in individuals who eat a low fat diet. Neither vitamin

D nor protein deficiency presents as a nutritional deficiency but as illness and disease.

The most common reasons cited for vitamin D deficiency is due to the lack of adequate sunlight exposure needed for vitamin D synthesis. Although this is true in theory, I think the high prevalence of vitamin D deficiency points to factors beyond the lack of sun exposure. Individuals who are able to synthesize vitamin D are really "ideal healthy individuals." Unfortunately, there are not as many of these types of people today as there were in the past. I believe there is another reason for the increased prevalence of vitamin D deficiency.

The real reason why individuals who have adequate sunlight exposure, yet cannot synthesize vitamin D, is because their skin cannot do so. The skin's decreased vitamin D synthesis ability is due to the lack of adequate nutrients. Nutritional deficiencies will affect your skin's ability to synthesize vitamin D just as it can affect the quality of your skin as you age. If you are deficient in protein, vitamins, minerals, and/or the essential fatty acids known as omega-3s, this will affect your skin's integrity. The reasons your skin wrinkles as you age are not due to aging but due to nutritional deficiencies and too much sun exposure. Vitamin D deficiency and its impact on health are unrealized and unappreciated.

The chance that your nutrition is optimal is dependent on what you have done right in regards to nutrition, up to this point in time. The truth is, your body still functions even if nothing is perfect or optimal. Your body has the advantage of calling upon the protein you already possess in the form of muscles and connective tissues if your daily consumption of the needed amino acids is deficient.

This is where your nutritional baseline matters, as this will determine how you are able to cope with current and future deficiencies. The disadvantage of calling upon your muscles and connective tissues as a resource pool is that the deficiencies of needed nutrients are not recognized. The outcome? Individuals will lose muscle mass and connective tissues over time. The loss of muscle mass and connective tissues are not the normal process of aging; they are signs of protein malnutrition.

Your body can use any of the macronutrients; sugars, fats and proteins as fuel. However, when you consume most of your calories in the form of sugars and fats, your body will begin to break down tissues composed of proteins. This is why your muscles are not able to maintain their size, no matter how hard you work out, if your daily protein intake is inadequate. The nutrient that keeps your body healthy is protein.

Proteins are the most essential building blocks for your body. Once a deficiency in protein or any of the other nutrients begin, the likelihood that it will worsen over time until a critical or tipping point event happens. At this point, a disease will develop. The speed and time of when a nutritional deficiency becomes critical is unknown due to variability in lifestyle and dietary intake. The reason why tipping points arise to cause an illness or disease is from a sudden increase in demand against the background of a limited nutritional baseline.

Stress: The Burden that It Places on Your Body's Nutritional Reserves

In life, we each have our own stressors that we have to deal with daily. Life's stressors are unavoidable and unpredictable in timing and severity. However, the combination of timing, duration and severity of daily stressors determine how deficient you can get in terms of your nutritional reservoir. Stressors can use up your body's nutrients just as if someone had stepped on a car's accelerator and used up the gasoline at a faster rate. Once your body is deficient of needed nutrients, it is set up for illness and disease. Events like this then just seem to happen "out of the blue." Yet, the truth is that your health does not just turn for the worse due to your age or a specific event. Illnesses and diseases are the cumulative effects of nutritional deficiencies occurring over time that lead to illness.

From the above discussion, illnesses and diseases are now explainable in individuals that are undergoing extreme periods of stress, such as the sudden onset of depression in an individual who had everything but then suddenly lost it all. You can say that the stress of extreme loss brought out an underlining subclinical family predisposition toward depression. Yes, an undiagnosed or predisposition for depression can contribute to the problem, but this explanation does not explain how the stressors brought about this disorder. Whether it is this example or something else that you might be familiar with, there are without a doubt, times when the health condition of an individual changes after an acute life stressor.

The amounts of protein needed daily increase in situations such as infection, injury, or other instances of increased bodily demand. For example, during the stress from severe infection or burns, the required daily protein intake increases from 0.8 grams to 1.5 gram or 2 gram per kilogram per day. A question to ask is "do we ever consider recommending a person to increase their daily protein intake as a way to deal with others stressors beyond burns or infection?" Would it not make sense that there are other stressful events in which a person's bodily demands for protein should be increased?"

Routinely, it is not considered normal practice to recommend people to increase their daily protein intake as a way to deal with life's stressors outside of a medical condition. I think it is time to reconsider the possibility that the current RDA requirement of 0.8 gram of protein per kilogram or 0.37 gram of protein per pound per day is exceedingly low. *I believe one reason that individuals are "aging," with chronic medical diseases, is due to an inadequate intake of daily protein throughout their lifetime.* Examples of two diseases that I believe are due to specific micro and macronutrient malnutrition are Parkinson's and Alzheimer's diseases. The specific micro and macronutrient deficiencies that may help cause Parkinson's and Alzheimer's disease are discussed later.

The tipping points are points in time where illnesses or diseases will result from nutritional deficiencies. This does not necessarily guarantee that the individual's health will inevitably spiral downward. Tipping point events are reversible if the causes are recognized. However, if nutritional deficiencies are not recognized, the likelihood for the deteriorating health is usually the case. Most of the time, the inciting factors leading to the tipping point are never changed. To reverse the tipping point, one has to recognize the importance of proper nutrition in health. For example, a person with Parkinson's disease, who has dysphasia (difficulty in swallowing), may aspirate when he eats, will likely go on to develop worsening malnutrition. Increased malnutrition will complicate his nutritional status and therefore cause his health to go into a downwards spiral. Any dietary changes or improvements to reduce existing stressors will help because it will help keep the body from raiding its limited nutritional supply. In this way, your body is better able to fend off debilitating stress. These are the reasons why an improvement in your diet or lifestyle after an illnesses or disease can help to improve your health.

Two examples of the ill effects of stressors-- one physical and the other psychological -- are used to highlight this point. For the synthesis of vitamin D, sunlight exposure is essential. However, exposing your skin to the sun's ultraviolet rays can cause skin damage since sunlight is a form of radiation. Exposure to radiation damages the cells in your body. Overexposing your skin to the sun's ultraviolet rays and your chances of skin wrinkles increase beyond what is expected for your age. The cause for premature skin wrinkling is simple. Premature wrinkling occurs when the ability for your body to repair and or replace the damaged skin cells is impaired. The impairment is secondary to a nutritional deficiency of the needed micro and macronutrients required for cellular repair.

Another case of premature aging occurs in individuals under stress such as public officials. An example is that of the Presidents of the United States of America or any high profile public servant. You can usually see premature aging in the form of graying of the hair color during their tenures in office. The etiology of premature aging such as hair graying is unknown. However, I believe that the etiology of a sun tanner's wrinkling skin and the graying of one's hair is the same. Premature aging is the result of nutritional deficiencies brought about by the increased physical or mental stress placed upon an individual. Individuals who are nutritionally insufficient or deficient do not have the nutritional reserve needed to maintain the metabolic demand put upon their body by the stressors. Once the stressors lessen, the aging from the nutritional malnutrition will stabilize but not necessarily reverse. Thus, the individual will not get back to the same condition as he once was before the stressors.

The statistics regarding the prevalence of stress in the United States are revealing. A telephone Gallup's poll of 1010 people taken in December 2006, found that more than 3 out of 4 Americans polled said they sometimes experience stress in their daily life, including roughly 4 out of 10 who experience it "frequently." Overall, the rates of reported stress levels have not changed much; from 1994, between 33% and 42% of Americans have reported frequently feeling stress. Only one in five individuals polled said that they are rarely stressed.

In addition, only 3% say they are never stressed. The following is the reported frequency of reported stress among individual age groups: 44% of 18- to 29-year-olds, 46% of 30- to 49-year-olds, 47% of parents with children under 18, 43% of full-time workers and 46% of part-time workers. Forty percent of women reported experiencing stress, compared to 35% of men. More than half of those polled -- 55% -- say they do not have enough time to do things they want to do.

These statistics point out how "stressed out" most people feel. Since there are so many people who feel that they are stressed, what can these individual do to help themselves deal with their daily stressors? The best way would be to eliminate or decrease the sources of stress. Another way, which is rarely considered, is for these individuals to increase their nutritional intake to meet the increased daily demand from their stressful lives.

Homeostasis (Equilibrium or Balance)

Homeostasis is defined as "the property of an open system, especially living organisms, to regulate its internal environment to maintain a stable, constant condition, by means of multiple dynamic equilibrium adjustments, controlled by interrelated regulation mechanisms." To achieve optimal health and vitality, your body's metabolic processes must be in a state of homeostasis, or equilibrium.

To be in homeostasis when all nutritional requirements are met is much less stressful on your body than if it had to obtain homeostasis from "multiple dynamic equilibrium adjustments, controlled by interrelated regulation mechanisms." Your ability to provide your body with the needed micro and macronutrients will affect how you are able to regulate your "internal environment to maintain a stable, constant condition."

Optimal heath is dependent on certain internal and external factors that are important for metabolism. Internal factors that affect your metabolism are in part genetically determined. How well your "organ systems" are functioning is in part genetically determined; for example. Genetic factors are things out of your control.

External factors that affect your metabolism include your environment. Environmental factors that have a negative effect on your metabolism are malnutrition, toxins, and injury. The environmental factor you have the most control over is your diet. The foods you choose to eat daily determine the health of your "organ system." This in turn determines your metabolism and the things that keep you healthy. From this perspective, your external nutritional environment governs your "organ system," and determines the potential for homeostasis. In fact, nutrition plays a greater role in your health and well-being than genetic factors. Dr. Francis Collins, the NIH's chief of genetics, states, *"Genes load the gun and the environment pulls the trigger."* I agree with this assessment.

In fact, each of us has a unique personality that is shaped by genetics and the surrounding environment. On a genetic level, I can say without a doubt that each of my daughters has unique personality traits of me and of their mother. These personality traits appear to have been genetically inherited rather than arising from learned environmental experiences. Nevertheless, your environmental experiences will influence and shape you to become the unique person you are. They will shape your overall personality possibly more than your genetic makeup. As such, no one else can ever have the same exact overall personality as you. Similarly, the nutrition you receive from the environment plays more of a critical role in your health than does your genetic make-up.

The reason to achieve optimal health is that it gives you the greatest chances to minimize illness and disease. Consider it as a state of health where you can be "all you can be" if your desire is for health and vitality. This is a state of health each of us can achieve with continual effort.

It is possible, through optimal nutrition, for your body's internal metabolism to be at homeostasis. This is the key to health because it reflects a state of internal balance. Balance, equilibrium, and homeostasis are all different words for the same principle. Any attempt to achieve optimal health and vitality must include this essential principle. *Optimal, balanced nutrition – defined as providing your body with the right balance of micronutrients and macronutrients that it needs daily – is the key to maintaining your body in homeostasis.*

Thousands upon thousands of persons have studied disease. Almost no one has studied health.

– Adelle Davis

Truth #7

The Clinical Importance of Nutrition

I am at a critical crossroad in my discussion about nutrition. That crossroad is in part due to me trying to convince you that improper nutrition or malnutrition is the cause for illnesses and diseases. Malnutrition often refers to a condition caused by deficiency in food calories needed to maintain health. This type of malnutrition is evident in situations where individuals simply do not have enough food to eat. At its worst, it is called starvation.

The term malnutrition I am referring to is not about food calories. It is less obvious, therefore not visibly recognized. It is about improper nutrition due to imbalances of the needed micro and macronutrients. This type of malnutrition is happening in our "modern day" society that has plenty of food calories to eat but lacks the proper food nutrients. This kind of malnutrition is not only about deficiencies but also about an over abundance of macronutrients. If malnutrition is causing illness and disease, then the way to health is by recognizing the nutrients needed and how one goes about getting enough of them. When I say proper nutrition is the answer to improve your health, my patients also agree.

The question you might want to ask is, "How and what evidence do I have that proper nutrition will work?" As to the "how" part of nutrition improving health, hopefully I have already given you some answers. For the evidence regarding nutrition and health, I will give examples of medical diagnoses where even though the etiologies to the causes are unknown, the answer might lie with malnutrition. Instead of looking at random diagnoses, I will look at the current top causes of human death in the United

States for 2006 and explain how they stem from improper nutrition.

The fifteen leading causes of death in 2006:

- Diseases of heart (heart disease)
- Malignant neoplasms (cancer)
- Cerebrovascular diseases (stroke)
- Chronic lower respiratory diseases
- Accidents (unintentional injuries)
- Diabetes mellitus (diabetes)
- Alzheimer's disease
- Influenza and pneumonia
- Nephritis, nephrotic syndrome and nephrosis (kidney disease)
- Septicemia
- Intentional self-harm (suicide)
- Chronic liver disease and cirrhosis
- Essential hypertension and hypertensive renal disease (hypertension)
- Parkinson's disease
- Assault (homicide)

If you eliminate accidents, self-harm, and assaults from the lists above, the causes left are really due to improper nutrition. The causes of these diagnoses are unknown. Yet, the diagnoses of cardiovascular diseases, cancers, diabetes, Alzheimer's disease, Parkinson's disease and infectious disease are causally linked to imbalances of needed micronutrients and macronutrients.

Recent evidence is pointing to the fact that human diseases are really due to cellular inflammation. Diseases associated with cellular inflammations are cardiovascular diseases, atherosclerosis, and autoimmune diseases. Evidence for cellular inflammation is from biomarkers of inflammation, detected by blood tests showing elevated C-reactive protein, sedimentation rate, and homocysteine. (*I believe total cholesterol and LDL are cardiovascular risk factors since they are really biomarkers of cellular inflammation.*) C-reactive protein (CRP) levels are high in cardiovascular diseases and in infections. The sedimentation rate is high in arthritis diseases, autoimmune disease, and again, infections. Similarly, an elevated homocysteine level is common in some individual with cardiovascular diseases.

The association between cellular inflammation and its relationship to human diseases is unknown. The current assumption in the management of diseases with elevated biomarkers of inflammation is that by lowering the abnormal biomarkers values, one can lower the risk of the diseases associated with the elevated levels. For instance, since homocysteine or C-reactive protein (CRP) is elevated in cardiovascular disease, by lowering homocysteine or CRP, this should lower cardiovascular disease risk. However, this assumption is false, since it is based on the false premise that treating biomarkers of inflammation will treat those conditions (diseases).

However, cellular inflammation and human diseases are explainable if you consider the following points. We know that cellular inflammation occurs as a normal process of homeostasis. Homeostasis encompasses all the metabolic processes needed to keep you alive and safeguard you from an ever-changing environment. The reasons cellular inflammation happens are best explained by looking at the mechanism of how your body defends itself against toxins, infections, cellular damage and foreign "invaders." By foreign invaders, I mean anything that your body recognizes as "not self," such as a transplanted organ. Cellular inflammation is by design a sign that your immune system is activated. This becomes detrimental for health when the process of acute cellular inflammation becomes chronic cellular inflammation. The mechanisms for illnesses or diseases are then due to uncontrollable acute or chronic cellular inflammation. The reason why acute or chronic cellular inflammation becomes uncontrollable is then the answer to illnesses or diseases.

Your immune system functions by two mechanisms: innate immune response and adaptive immune response. The innate immune response, also known as your humeral immune system, is evolutionarily ancient and found in all multi-cellular eukaryotic organisms. The adaptive or cellular immunity is present in higher organisms such as vertebrates. Your immune systems function to protect you against toxins, infections and in the regulatory process of cell repair. In these aspects, your immune system acts as a homeostatic system; its main function is to first protect you against what are foreign to your body. Its second function is more of a "housekeeping" function, which is to help restore cellular balance.

When looking at the causes of illnesses and diseases, keep these points in mind. Health and vitality are possible when your body is at homeostasis, or equilibrium. Homeostasis is a state of balance and a state your body prefers to keep you in at all times.

Any factors that knock you out of homeostasis are not welcomed.

Factors that affect homeostasis are either extrinsic or intrinsic. Extrinsic factors include toxins, infections, injuries, and most importantly nutrition. These factors are your external environment. Intrinsic factors are found within your body. The intrinsic factor affecting homeostasis is your genetic make-up.

The most important factor, since it determines how well your body is able to respond to other extrinsic factors, is your nutrition. A balanced and adequate nutritional eating pattern is your key to health and vitality. The factor with adverse health consequences is malnutrition. When malnutrition occurs, your body is not in homeostasis. This is when a state of acute pathologic or acute adaptive inflammation occurs. Your body's ability to handle this situation will determine if homeostasis resumes toward a balanced state. Otherwise, chronic inflammation, illnesses, and diseases ensue due to those adaptive measures your body has to undergo to cope with the internal and external environments. Acute pathologic or adaptive inflammation that is not resolved causes illnesses.

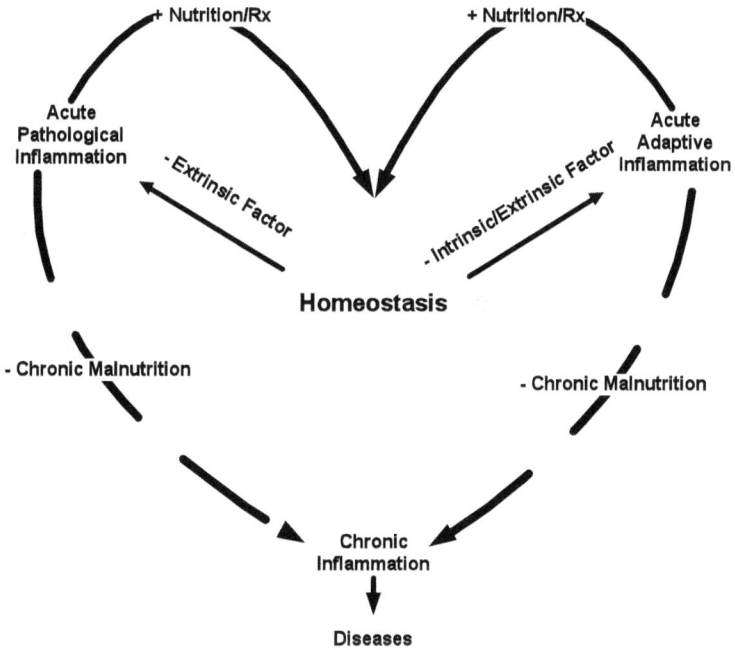

+ Nutrition/Rx   + Nutrition/Rx

Acute   Acute
Pathological   Adaptive
Inflammation   Inflammation

- Extrinsic Factor   - Intrinsic/Extrinsic Factor

Homeostasis

- Chronic Malnutrition   - Chronic Malnutrition

Chronic
Inflammation

Diseases

Intrinsic factor: Genetics

Extrinsic factor: Environmental (infection; toxin; injury; nutrition)

Cardiovascular Disease

The most common cause of human mortality in 2006 was cardiovascular diseases. Besides death, the co-morbidities from cardiovascular disease and the economic costs associated with it are enormous. The risk factors for cardiovascular disease are obesity, hypertension, hyperlipidemia, and diabetes.

However, the risks factors associated with cardiovascular diseases do not explain its etiology but are just an association. In fact, the etiologies of the risk factors are themselves a mystery. Nevertheless, the causes for cardiovascular diseases or any diseases are explainable if you have an open mind and start by looking at nutrition, since this is the basis of what is keeping you alive. By examining the different diet patterns that exist today, what you can see are diet patterns that are based on ease of production. They are delivered and packaged for convenience but are not beneficial for your health since they are not balanced in any of the nutrients that are needed by your body to function properly. As a result, what you end up with is an imbalanced diet pattern that leads directly to cardiovascular diseases and illnesses.

The general diet pattern most prevalent today consists of processed foods. These foods are imbalanced in the macronutrients and deficient in the micronutrients. Processed foods such as pre-packaged foods or fast foods regulated by the USDA are low in protein and high in carbohydrate.

A diet pattern low in protein and high in carbohydrate is identifiable by comparing the carbohydrate to protein ratio (CP ratio). Comparing the total grams of carbohydrate to the total grams of protein in a serving size will yield the CP ratio. A low fat diet pattern is identifiable by a high carbohydrate to protein ratio (CP ratio), often in the ratio of 6:1 to 10:1. Processed foods and fast foods are high in refined carbohydrates, added sugars, and are very often low in proteins.

A low fat diet pattern is the recommended diet pattern that most individuals are following if they have hyperlipidemia or want to avoid cardiovascular disease. A low fat diet pattern, the USDA food pyramid, and the Daily Values, all represent the same diet that is high in carbohydrates and low on proteins. The irony about following this type of diet, as I've mentioned, is that it will predispose you to have the very thing you are trying to avoid: obesity, hyperlipidemia, heart diseases, hypertension, and stroke. *Believe me, the low fat diet pattern that you are eating is causing those diseases you are trying to avoid.*

Since the 1970's, the diet-heart paradigm goes something like this: a high dietary intake of saturated fat and cholesterol increases the risk of atherosclerosis and ischemic heart disease (IHD). Believing that dietary fat is the cause for hyperlipidemia, atherosclerosis and ischemic heart disease (IHD) led the USDA to recommend and promote a low fat dietary pattern as a way to prevent IHD. However, a low fat diet pattern is typically low in fat and low in protein while high in refined carbohydrates and sweetener such as high fructose corn syrup.

The shift in the eating habits from eating animal products to a low fat diet pattern is contributing to a lower intake of dietary protein and essential fats. Eating too much carbohydrate -- which prompts your liver to produce too much cholesterol and triglycerides -- and not enough dietary proteins and unsaturated fats are the main reasons for atherosclerosis and ischemic heart disease (IHD).

Another way to look for possible causes of cardiovascular disease is to look for known diseases associated with heart disease, strokes, and hypertension. As it turns out to be, there is one such disease associated with all three. This disease is call fibromuscular dysplasia, a disease that affects one or more arteries in the body.

Leadbetter and Burkland first observed fibromuscular dysplasia (FMD) in 1938 in a 5-year-old boy that had renal (kidney) disease. The arteries affected in FMD are medium to large sized, such as renal arteries, coronary arteries, pulmonary arteries, and the aorta. The pathologic defect seen in FMD typically develops in the arterial wall and present clinically as narrowing or dilation within the vessel walls. Radiographic finding of FMD have a "string of beads" appearance. Individuals who have FMD will have symptoms related to the location of the affected arteries. When the renal arteries are involved, you can have high blood pressure from renal artery stenosis. Renal atrophy or renal failure can also occur. When the carotid arteries are involved, symptoms such as dizziness, headache, and ringing in the ears can occur. Fibromuscular dysplasia (FMD) diseases of the carotid arteries cause transient ischemic attack and strokes from intracranial aneurysms. Therefore, diseases associated with FMD are heart disease, hypertension, and stroke.

The etiology of FMD is unknown but genetic inheritance could play a causal role. Other possible causes associate with FMD includes tobacco use, changes in estrogen level, and ischemia from abnormal vessel development. These potential causes can indeed be a true association, yet I believe that a better explanation exists. I believe the actual cause for FMD is due to acute and chronic blood vessel inflammation secondary to a lifetime of protein and essential fatty acid malnutrition.

The effects of protein and essential fatty acid malnutrition explain the etiology of FMD better then that currently exists. Arteries are made-up of three layers of muscles along with other connective tissues. Muscles and connective tissues are made-up of proteins. Arteries are blood vessels that carry blood away from the heart and as such are under higher pressure than the venous system. The pressure from the pumping action of the heart will cause blood to flow, and with that flow, there will be potential for the cells lining the inner walls of the blood vessels to be damaged over time. The pressure and flow of blood will cause normal wear and tear on the vessel walls and with it the need for those cells to be repaired. The ability for your body to repair and maintain the integrity of the cells that line the inner vessel wall should be automatic. However, not everything that happens automatically will, if your nutritional statuses are compromised.

The adverse health effect due to heart diseases and stroke is the result of ischemia. Ischemia is the result of atherosclerosis or plaque rupture with emboli that cause vessel obstruction and myocardial infarction. In the heart, myocardial cells are damaged from ischemia either alone or in concert with hypertension. The result is congestive heart failure. In the brain, neuronal cells death occurs from ischemia due to a blocked carotid atherosclerosis, embolic or from a hemorrhagic caused by an aneurysm. Heart disease and strokes share similar etiology of atherosclerosis and plaque rupture. Thus, if you can explain the cause for atherosclerosis and plaque rupture, you can then identify a preventable cause for both.

The causes for atherosclerosis are multi-factorial. One condition speculated to be the cause for atherosclerosis is hyperlipidemia or high blood cholesterol. Having high blood cholesterols as a cause for atherosclerosis is true for only those few individuals who have a genetic condition where there is a defect in the LDL cholesterol transport. However, most individuals do not have a genetic susceptibility for hyperlipidemia and thus a dietary factor may be to blame.

Your body is able to regulate the biosynthesis of fats from your liver depending on a number of factors. The stimulus for the endogenous biosynthesis of cholesterol are: 1) on an as- needed basis depending on dietary cholesterol intake, 2) on an as-needed basis depending on cellular damage, 3) dependent on total caloric intake from either carbohydrate or protein. What "on an as-needed" basis means is that your body self- regulates its own cholesterol by the presence of the level of cholesterol in your bloodstream. High blood cholesterol from a higher dietary intake of fatty foods would lead to a net decrease in endogenous cholesterol production. A lower dietary intake of cholesterol will stimulate your liver for endogenous cholesterol biosynthesis. The regulatory mechanism for the biosynthesis of cholesterol starts within the endoplasmic reticulum (ER) of your cells. Protein synthesis by your ER is how your body is able to detect the cholesterol level. Your body will also need to increase cholesterol biosynthesis as a normal process in homeostasis to repair damaged cells. When there are cellular injuries, the biosynthesis of cholesterol from your liver will increase since the cell's bi-lipid layer membrane has cholesterol molecules within it. Atherosclerosis is believed to be cause by hyperlipidemia. However, could the hyperlipidemia associated with atherosclerosis be really from a reactive inflammatory reaction of cellular damage that is driving up the endogenous biosynthesis of cholesterol from your liver?

Your body's ability to self-regulate the biosynthesis of cholesterol from dietary cholesterol intake make recommending a low fat dietary pattern the wrong advice for treating hyperlipidemia. Maybe eating a low fat diet is not such a good idea in trying to lower hyperlipidemia. In fact, most individuals who believe that a low fat diet pattern is the healthy way to eat do not realize that it is really a high carbohydrate diet pattern, i.e. sugar. A high carbohydrate diet is detrimental for health for these reasons: It stimulates insulin secretion and action for energy metabolism. With excess consumption of carbohydrate, carbohydrates are first used and those that are not used initially are stored as glycogen and then as fats. Before sugars become fats in your adipose tissues, the sugars are synthesized into triglycerides. Hypertriglyceridemia is the result of your liver's endogenous fats synthesis from eating too many carbohydrates.

Another reason why eating carbohydrate is detrimental for health is that when you are eating carbohydrates, you are not eating enough dietary fats to prevent endogenous cholesterols synthesis from occurring. Not eating enough dietary fats will also result in not getting enough dietary proteins. A low dietary fat and protein intake causes an imbalanced diet pattern and therefore leads to malnutrition of proteins and essential fats. Malnutrition of cholesterol and non-essential fats does not occur since you can endogenously synthesize them.

Cancer

Cancer was the second leading cause of death, behind cardiovascular disease, in the United States in 2006. If we are able to understand what causes cardiovascular disease and cancer, we would be able to prevent the deaths associated with it and many of its co-morbidities and health related costs.

In 2009, approximately 1,479,350 new cases of cancer were diagnosed and accounted for about 562,340 deaths. We currently know that cancer is due to a single human cell that is able to divide uncontrollably. The ability for a single cell to divide uncontrollably is not a characteristic found in normal cells. Cancer cells are usually of somatic cell origin and not from a germ cell line. All cells in your body are somatic cells except for those cells that make up the sperm or egg cells. A cancer cell is not transmittable from one generation to the next or inherited since most cancer originates from somatic cells. The only way cancer passes from one generation to the next is if a mutation occurs in the gonads or is within the genome from gonad cells.

Cancer usually starts out as a single somatic cell that grows uncontrollably due to an abnormal regulatory cell cycle that would normally control cell division. The reason for the uncontrolled growth of a cancer cell could be due to a mutation within its cell cycle regulatory mechanism. Normal cell division occurs through an orderly process known as the cell cycle. The cell cycle has four major active phases and one inactive phase. The active phases are the G1, S, G2 and mitosis. The inactive resting phase of the cell cycle is call the G0 phase. The regulatory point in the cell cycle that controls whether cell division proceeds or stops is at the end of the G1 phase. The regulatory point at the end of G1 phase that controls cell division is called the restriction point or R point. The restriction point is the critical point in the cell cycle that regulates cell division. When this restriction point regulatory process fails, normal cells become cancerous.

Normal cells will go through the process of cell division when they have the right stimulus to do so. The stimuli for cell division are from growth factors. Growth factors stimulate cells to divide as part of the normal repair process from cells damaged from local injury or from environmental toxin. The way that cancer can arise, from a normal cell, is when the normal homeostatic process of the restriction point regulatory process in a cell cycle goes awry. Normally, a cell will cycle through the different phases of cell division and then will stop dividing by exiting the cell cycle. It will then proceed to the G0 phase. Cell division needs to be regulated since if it was not; you would have more cells than you actually need to replace "aged" or damaged cells. In order for the cells in your body to function as part of a tissue system and organ system, cell division needs to be highly regulated.

For instance, when you have an injury such as a cut on your arm, your body is able to heal itself with the exact precision needed to replace only those damaged cells. Apoptosis, a process that govern cell death, is part of the normal cell cycle that your body uses to maintain a balanced number of cells in your body. This is part of the larger homeostatic mechanism that your body has in place to maintain cellular order.

Cancer is due to an abnormal cellular regulatory process in which cancer cells continue to divide when cell division should have stopped. Normal cells, when put into a Petri dish with the proper nutrients and growth factor, will divide and form a single monolayer of cells. When these normal cells touch each other, further cell proliferation and division stops. Normal cells exhibit contact inhibition. Cancer cells lack contact inhibition and are able keep on dividing. They are also able to produce their own growth factors. When this happens, there are more cells in a tissue or organ then there should be. Cancer cells are able to divide and will keep on dividing uncontrollably.

If this increased cell division continues, it can cause a mass effect due to the increased number of cells presented in a tissue or organ. The mass effect from the cancer cell does not cause death in the individuals. In fact, most cancers do not grow to the point of causing a cell mass problem and therefore do not explain why cancer cells cause death. Even with the greater number of cells in a tissue or organ, your body does not react against it through inflammation. The reason inflammation does not occur is because the cancer cells are your own cells and are not initially recognized as foreign. As such, the inflammatory reaction seen as a defensive mechanism for foreign agents is not stimulated.

Your body functions as a very efficient "machine," when given the chance. What this means is when provided with the micro and macronutrients needed, your body will function as it should, efficiently and in an orderly fashion. When the micro and macronutrients environment is imbalanced or inadequate to provide your body with what it needs, your body will have to adapt to the situation and function sub-optimally. The goal ultimately is to maintain internal homeostasis. Your body has the mechanisms in place to keep you alive and functioning optimally. Cell division occurs in an orderly fashion since there are internal control systems in place to make sure this happens. However, things do not always work out this way since nutritionally, malnutrition is a real problem that your body has to deal with everyday. A suboptimal condition like malnutrition is how I believe cancer can arise since cell division requires the precision not afforded by an imbalance or inadequate micro and macronutrient environment.

Your body goes through about 10,000,000,000,000,000 cells division in your lifetime. This number works to be about 10,000,000 cells division in a second. This many cells going through cell division would require all processes to work accordingly. Malnutrition can make cell division go awry and can set the stage for cancer to occur. It leads your body to adapt to a suboptimal nutritional environment. Cell division requires an optimal nutritional environment so that the cell cycles function properly by having the building blocks needed. However, when the nutritional environment is suboptimal, this leads a single normal cell to be transformed into a mutant cell. A mutant cell will break away from the normal cell cycle process as a mechanism of adaptation.

Other obstacles in normal cell function are external factors such as cellular damage caused by physical injuries, toxins, and infections. Physical injuries caused increased cellular division to repair those cells that are damaged. Toxins or infections are any substances living or foreign to your body and are from the external environment. For instance, if your body detects something foreign, your immune system will mount an inflammatory reaction to fight against the foreign object or agent. The reason why a transplanted organ is rejected by your body is because of your innate immune system defending against an organ perceived as foreign. Controlling the inflammatory reaction that results from injuries or infections are part of the treatment regimen of many diseases.

The treatments modalities currently used to treat most cancer depend on the location of the cancer and its tissue type. One treatment modality is surgery: This is the most direct and specific in the sense that it is removing the cancer cells by cutting them out. However, this method is not always possible due to either location, size or because the cancer cells have already metastasized. The second method in which cancer cell death can occur is through chemotherapy. This method is based on using the differences between the cell replication processes of cancer cells versus normal cells. Fast dividing cancer cells are killed by chemotherapy while normal replicating cells are less likely to be killed. The third treatment modality is radiation. This is the nonspecific method of killing cancer cells by using radiation. The use of radiation to treat cancer is like trying to get rid of an insect on the leaf of the plant by spraying insecticide specifically on that insect while it is on the leaf. Spraying the insecticide will kill the insect but might also kill the surrounding tissues of the plant. These treatment modalities are often used in combination, with each having its positive and negative effects.

If you are wondering about the actual mechanisms that individuals with cancer die from, I do not believe we know the answers. You can say that cancers kill, but to say they kill without knowing the actual mechanism makes cancer death that more difficult to circumvent. I will try to speculate as to the mechanism of how cancers kill. One possible explanation as to how cancer cells can kill an individual is if the cancer cells somehow produce a chemical or substance that is toxic to life. This explanation, however, does not seem to fit our current understanding of the differences between cancer cells and normal cells. Cancer is usually due to a single somatic cell that is able to divide uncontrollably. The definition that I found on Wikipedia for cancer is: "Cancer is a class of diseases or disorders characterized by uncontrolled division of cells and the ability of these cells to invade other tissues, either by direct growth into adjacent tissue through invasion, or by implantation into distant sites by metastasis."

This is the widely held definition for cancer no matter where you look. An important point within that definition that I have not pointed out before but need to emphasize is, "the ability of these cells to invade other tissues, either by direct growth into adjacent tissue through invasion, or by implantation into distant sites." The ability to metastasize is what separates abnormally dividing cells from being classified as either benign or cancerous. A cell whose cell division is abnormal does not itself make it cancerous.

For example, psoriasis is a chronic skin disease that affects about 4.5 million individuals in the United States. The cause is due to an immune-mediated reaction. The defect in psoriasis is due to a defect in the body's immune system that causes the body to over-react and accelerate the growth of skin cells. Normal skin cells mature and shed from the skin's surface every 28 to 30 days. In psoriasis, this process occurs in 3 to 6 days. With the shortened cycle, the skin cells pile up instead of being shed, causing the visible lesions. This example highlights the point that it is the metastasis potential of cancer cells that distinguishes whether uncontrolled cells division from a cancer cell will kill or not. Even with the requirement of metastasis, unless the cancer cells metastasize to a vital organ needed for survival, what is the actual mechanism of death?

I speculate that the reason cancer cells end up killing a person is due to your body's inability to maintain homeostasis. Death then is the body's way of trying to keep cancer cells from continuously growing uncontrollably. It could be that cancer causes death when the body is able to recognize the cancer cells as "abnormal." The cancer cells are not recognized as foreign due to their uncontrolled growth but due to their metastatic ability to spread to other areas of your body. Cancer cells are targeted as "foreign cells" by the immune system when they metastasize. When your body tries to mount an attack against these cancer cells is when it ultimately leads to the death of the individual.

In an article in Scientific America, dated January 10, 2007, the author and journalist Carl Zimmer, "Evolved for Cancer," theorized that cancer arises as part of the inevitable possibility that comes with the natural selection process. The way that I understood his theory is that during cell division copying errors in the genetic material will occur. Our cells are able to minimize DNA errors from occurring. However, errors will happen. It is from these DNA replication errors that lead to abnormal cellular growth, abnormal apoptosis, and this leads to cancer. In the natural selection process, some of these DNA copying errors are passed on from generation to generation. One reason most cancer occurs at the late stage of life is that the cells are efficient in replicating your genes without making any mistakes.

Carl Zimmer's view is that cancer can arise from some type of error that occurs during the gene duplication processes. I agree with this assessment. In fact, it is harder to imagine how a cell is able to perform all the needed cell function so perfectly. Carl Zimmer's article brings up an aspect of cancer as occurring due to error in the DNA replication processes that is highly regulated. Your body has the mechanism to prevent any error from occurring during the gene replication process. In fact, it is theorized that more cancers would be prevalent if your body did not have a way to prevent errors in the gene replication process from occurring.

The fact is that your body does have a mechanism to suppress cancer. The tumor suppressing protein called the p53 tumor suppression protein is one such mechanism. A gene mapped to chromosome 17 of your DNA codes the p53 protein. The function of this p53 gene is that it codes for a protein whose activity stops the formation of tumors. Individuals who inherit only one functional copy of this p53 gene from their parents are predisposed to certain cancers. The Li-Fraumeni syndrome is an example of cancer occurring in a variety of tissues in early adulthood. Through the billions of years of natural selection, your internal mechanism for regulation of homeostasis will also prevent cancers from occurring. The possible explanation as to the cause of death for individuals with cancer is the result of your body's homeostatic mechanism recognizing that there are cells that lack cell regulation and have metastasized.

Obesity and Diabetes

After cardiovascular diseases and cancer, diabetes ranks as a leading cause of mortality. The top leading risk factor for diabetes is obesity. In fact, diseases that often co-exist with obesity ("co-morbidities" in doctor speak) include coronary heart disease, hypertension, stroke, and certain types of cancer. Understanding the natural history of how an individual can become obese will enable us to decrease the prevalence of coronary heart disease, hypertension, stroke, and diabetes morbidity and mortality.

It is a fact that obesity is at an epidemic level in the United States. Recent statistic points out that one out of four American are obese while three out of four are overweight; with overweight defined by a BMI 25 or greater. Obesity is not just isolated here in the USA but is becoming an increasingly global problem. The reasons why an individual becomes obese are many, debatable, and still not fully understood. At this time, I will give my opinion as to why the rate of obesity is on the rise. I will begin by discussing the mechanisms behind weight gain leading to obesity.

Factors that determine or affect your metabolism will determine your weight. In nutrition, traditional weight loss methods are based on cutting calories. In theory, as long as you reduce your total daily caloric intake, you will lose weight. Total daily caloric intake affecting body weight can be considered the calories in, calories out principle. Simply stated, the more calories you eat, the greater chances you will gain weight over time. Conversely, the less you eat, the greater chances you will lose weight over time. This sounds reasonable, and guess what? It is true.

Yet, there are opponents that believe that the total calories do not matter. They believe that the calories do not matter since weight gain is simply due to a process of fat or adipose tissue accumulation. To them, that is the cause of obesity. Eating foods that stimulate this process -- too many carbohydrates, they believe, causes you to accumulate fat.

The notion of consuming excessive carbohydrate calories as driving fat accumulation is true. However, consuming too many calories from either proteins or fats will also cause your body to gain weight via fat accumulation. *Obesity will happen if you consume too many calories, and this occurs even if those calories are from proteins or fats.*

In individuals that are able to lose weight and maintain the weight loss, the "calories in, calories out" principle invariably explains some of the reasons behind the weight loss. Consuming fewer calories by portion control will work only if you are able to eat less than you did before.

Changing or eliminating certain macronutrients such as carbohydrates from your diet will also help you lose weight. Compared to eating carbohydrates, eating proteins and fats does help decrease appetite. The satiety factor due to the type of macronutrients you choose to eat is where proteins and fats have advantages over carbohydrates. However, realize that you cannot eat all the calories you want -- even in the form of proteins and fats -- if the total calories are greater than your metabolic requirement per day. You can reasonably calculate your daily caloric requirement by multiplying your body weight in pounds by 10 kcal to get your total daily caloric requirement. Eating more calories than needed, as calculated by one's metabolic requirement, is doomed to fail as evidenced by increasing weight.

The reasons why some individuals disbelieve the "calorie in, calorie out" principle are because they do not believe that your body treats foods calorie equally. The problem with this type of thinking is that they forget that a calorie is simply a measurement of energy. One fat calorie is equal to one carbohydrate calorie, which is equal to one protein calorie. This is indeed true and will always be true. However, even though the energy potential is similar for the individual macronutrient, the metabolism or health consequences are not equivalent. Each macronutrient exerts different health consequence depending if you consume too much or too little of the specific macronutrient. Fats and proteins are more "satisfying" metabolically, in the sense that one tends to eat less when a meal is composed of proteins or fats.

The opposite is true for the consumption of carbohydrates. Carbohydrate consumption causes increased insulin secretion and greater fluctuation in blood glucose level. Consuming too many carbohydrates will result in "sugar craving," and eventual weight gain and obesity. Over time, excessive carbohydrate consumption, as defined by total caloric consumption of over 70% of total daily caloric intake, will cause a vicious cycle of carbohydrate addiction-- i.e. "sweet tooth."

Another reason that obesity occurs is the result of your metabolism. I alluded to an individual's metabolism when I discussed macronutrients metabolism. Yet, an issue more central to weight regulation is your basal metabolic rate. Your basal metabolic rate is simply the amount of energy in Kilocalories needed to keep you alive. The classic equation used to determine your basal metabolic rate

(BMR) is the Harris-Benedict equation. To determine your total daily caloric need, you would multiple the BMR by an activity level. The amounts of energy required for cellular functions at any time depend on your basal metabolic rate (BMR) plus an activity factor. If you exercise and are physically active, this will keep your basal metabolic rate higher than if you are sedentary. Physical activity is comparable to stepping on a car's accelerator; this will speed up the engine and will burn off more energy then at basal metabolic rate.

Any factors or mechanisms that negatively influence your basal metabolic rate will make it difficult for you to metabolize the food calories consumed. Your total daily caloric need is what determines your daily energy requirement. When your metabolic rate increases, you will "burn" more calories at a faster rate then normally. Similarly, when your metabolic rate is reduced, fewer calories are used from the foods consumed and you will feel tired and sluggish. When you eat foods, the food calories are used to keep you alive. The food calories not used by cellular metabolism will be stored. Remember that for the most part, you do not store excessive food calories as glucose or proteins but as fats.

If you have more lean muscle mass than fat, your caloric demand will be higher then if you have less muscle mass. Muscle metabolic demand is higher than fat and thus your need of calories will continue throughout the day. Fat, on the other hand, has little metabolic demand for food calories. The benefit of having muscle mass over fat mass is that muscle uses energy while fat does not. This means that by increasing your muscle mass, you can actually increase your basal metabolic rate and thus your body will consume more food calories from your meal instead of having those calories be unused and stored as excessive fat. Fat essentially is stored energy and does not consume any calories.

A couple of factors determine your metabolic rate. How well you sleep, in the sense of quality and quantity, will affect your weight since sleep has an effect on your metabolism. A low functioning thyroid or a hyperactive thyroid will also affect your weight. Hypothyroidism will slow down your metabolic rate so that the foods ingested are metabolized incorrectly therefore leading to greater weight gains. Another factor determining your metabolic rate is the frequency of your meals. Occasionally skipping a few meals here and there will be fine, and will not reset your metabolic rate. However, continually skipping certain meals will cause a longer duration between meals and will adversely affect your body, causing it to have a slower metabolic rate. This is your body's adaptive homeostatic mechanism needed for survival during what your body perceives as starvation.

Everyone knows that eating breakfast is important. In fact, eating breakfast is essential for having a normal metabolic rate. If you skip breakfast, the duration between dinner and your next meal could be well in excess of twelve hours. The duration between meals, if you skip breakfast, makes your metabolism counterproductive to your overall weight. Not eating or feeding your body of the calories needed sends the wrong message and is detrimental to your metabolic rate. Long durations between meals will cause your basal metabolic rate to slow down to the minimal rate that will sustain you. The continuation of skipping breakfast or meals will escalate a cycle of lower basal metabolic rate and lower usage of digested calories and greater storage of those food calories consumed.

When you skip this important meal, in fact, you are essentially conveying an incorrect signal for your body to lower your metabolic rate to match the energy availability during starvation. With a lower metabolic rate, foods eaten are not metabolized properly and will instead be stored as fat. A person's overall weight is the result of how well they metabolize the foods consumed. An abnormal metabolic state such as that of "insulin resistance" can also affect a person's weight. (Remember that I have hypothesized that the mechanism for insulin resistance is due to vitamin D deficiency.)

The reason obesity is occurring is because of three independent and yet interrelated processes. The first is the calories in, calories out principle. The second reason for obesity is the type of calories consumed. The third reason for obesity is how your body deals with those macronutrient calories consumed via metabolism.

I believe that most overweight individuals are suffering from protein, vitamin, or mineral deficiencies. This may be due to the inadequate consumption of the amounts of nutrients needed for their specific weight and metabolic demands. In most cases, the importance of body weight is not used in the determination of the needed nutrients. But weight, along with an individual's metabolic rate, is an important factor that determines the individual daily nutritional needed. The metabolic rate of an individual is the result of the combined effects of both the basal and active metabolic rate.

Why Is It So Hard to Lose Weight?

Next, I would like to concentrate from a calorie standpoint as to why it is so hard to lose weight. As stated above, a person will not lose weight if they eat too much. Consuming more calories than needed, no matter what macronutrients, will cause weight gain.

The amount of calories that keeps you alive is your basal metabolic rate (BMR). A generic method to determine your BMR is by multiplying your body weight in kilogram by twenty kilocalories. For daily caloric need in pounds of body weight, you should multiply body weight in pounds by ten kilocalories. The number you get from using this simple equation is your BMR.

Your basal metabolic rate is the factor that determines the rate at which the food calories eaten are used. As such, an individual will not lose weight if his or her basal metabolic rate is counterproductive to burning the calories consumed. For instance, if your BMR is lower, instead of burning the food calories you are consuming, the calories will be stored. Therefore, the way to lose weight is to eat less or to increase your basal metabolic rate. This might sound simple yet is very difficult for most of us to achieve. Thus, the reason why individuals cannot lose weight is that their BMR is abnormally slow, and second, they are not able to eat less.

I have patients that would "swear" that they do not eat "anything" and yet they are not able to lose weight. They would say that they do not know why they cannot lose weight. Now you can see it is your BMR, which is counterproductive to your effort to lose weight.

The other reason why you cannot lose weight has to do with overeating. Excessive eating becomes such a routine that most people eat even when not hungry. Once a routine is developed, it becomes a need. This is when deviating from the routine becomes difficult.

The one thing that your body tries to maintain is your current body weight. Your body does not know what weight you should be. It just knows that to deviate from the current body weight is a change. Your body will maintain your current body weight by telling you when you are hungry and when to eat but not necessarily how much to eat. Most people will not stop eating when they are no longer hungry. They continue eating until they have overeaten and until they are absolutely stuffed. If you are able to stop eating before you have over eaten, then your weight will be stable. If you cannot break away from this cycle of over indulgence or snacking between meals, your body weight will increase. It will also start demanding a greater amount of calories than what it was requiring at your previous weight.

If you want to lose weight, you must cut back your total daily caloric intake or increase your basal metabolic rate. Decreasing caloric intake over an extended period is the difficult task required for sustained weight lost. Hunger is the reason why most people cannot stick to a plan of a lower caloric intake diet. Hunger is due to the natural sensation that one gets from either a lower caloric intake or perceived nutritional deficiencies. Hunger is the built in mechanism for survival. It is the signal you get when your body is running low on the calories and nutrients it needs to maintain your bodily functions. Hunger is the signal that tells you that you need to eat; however, there is no signal that will tell you what to eat.

The reason behind the recommendation for eating many small meals throughout the day is based on the fact of supplying your body with a "constant" calorie stream so that your metabolic rate stays steady and does not slow down. If you were to skip breakfast and the last meal was dinner, then over many weeks or months, your metabolic rate would down-regulate to match what the body is reacting to as a starved state. During a lowered basal metabolic rate state, not everything consumed will be used. Eating at regular intervals negates your body's perception of a decreased calorie state. This will result in a higher basal metabolic rate.

The macronutrient that tends to make a person over eat is the consumption of sugars. By sugars, I mean any foods that are carbohydrates. Sugar or glucose is a carbohydrate. However, one thing that most individuals do not realize is that starches from grains and wheat are also a carbohydrate. When you eat a fruit that taste sweet, realize it is glucose and fructose you are eating. The benefit of eating fruits and vegetables is due to their vitamins and minerals content. *Today, consuming fruits and vegetables will not provide you with the same amount of vitamins and minerals as it once did in the old farming days when the soil was more fertile.*

Also, the overconsumption of carbohydrates of any form is the cause for an imbalanced diet and is the driving force behind the sugar craving and sugar addiction. The explanation for the "sugar craving" that individuals who consume carbohydrates have is from the increase insulin release as a response to carbohydrates. Insulin released from carbohydrate consumption will lower your blood glucose. The decreased blood glucose will then trigger the hunger signal that then starts this whole cycle over again.

Another answer for the "sugar craving" is that when you are craving sweets, what your body is craving is not necessarily carbohydrates but the deficient nutrients from the foods eaten. When your body is deficient in a certain macronutrient, it does not have the capacity to say, feed me this deficient nutrient or that deficient nutrient. Your body cannot tell you which nutrients are deficient from your diet. The only signal that our body can give you is of hunger and thirst.

Hunger and thirst are your body's signal for food calories and water. However, hunger could also act as your body's signal to increase its chances of getting the needed nutrients via eating foods. Yet the foods that you tend to eat are those that you are accustomed to, foods that taste good or the ones that are readily available. Foods that fit this criteria are often either fast foods or processed foods. Fast foods or processed foods are there to provide food calories and are mostly carbohydrate-based type of foods. The differences between processed foods, whole foods or organic foods are their nutrient quality and quantity. Processed foods have less micronutrients such as vitamins and minerals and more macronutrients like carbohydrates. The reverse is true for eating whole or organic foods.

When looking at current weight loss recommendations, it is good to understand the rationale behind the mechanism of why they could or could not work. Exercise works in weight loss by increasing an individual's basal metabolic rate. This is the real reason why exercise can be effective as a weight loss method. However, I believe that except for a small number of individuals, weight loss does not occur from the calories lost from the exercise performed, but from the higher metabolic rate that the exercise can stimulate. With a higher metabolic rate, one is able to burn off the calories from the foods eaten.

Other benefits from exercise have to do with increasing lean muscle mass. Muscles are better than fats in that they will actually consume calories instead of acting as "dead weight" on your body. If you were able to burn more calories from the foods eaten, then there would be fewer calories left that your body would need to store. Weight loss is possible if you burn more calories than you consumed during the day. Exercising will not enable you to lose weight if your total caloric intake also increases. This is where the hidden or not so obvious calories that you consume, in the form of sport drinks or other health snacks are counterproductive in terms of weight loss.

The Hidden Costs of Too Many Carbs

The adverse health effects from the overconsumption of carbohydrates includes: central obesity as defined by increased waist circumference or BMI, high fasting plasma glucose, a high blood triglycerides, and low HDL. The interesting things about these factors are that they are the same factors that constitute "metabolic syndrome." Metabolic syndrome is a combination of medical disorders that increases the risk for developing cardiovascular disease and diabetes. Going back to the "calories in, calories out" principle of food nutrition, think about this equation being actually "calories in, metabolism, calories out." The overconsumption of carbohydrate is the "calories in" part of the equation. The metabolic syndrome is the "calories out." The missing link that really predisposes an individual to have metabolic syndrome is metabolism. Things that determine your metabolism are your body's basal metabolic rate, your activity level, and your vitamin D level. In my opinion, the single greatest risk factor for an abnormal metabolic state leading to metabolic syndrome and diabetes is vitamin D deficiency.

Obesity, integrally linked to Type 2 diabetes and hyperlipidemia, is also reasonably tied to vitamin D deficiency. Increasingly a worldwide concern is obesity. Worldwide, obesity is believed to result from a shift from a predominantly vegetarian to a high-calorie diet. Such high-calorie diets typically include beverages, such as soda and beer, which are high in calories, but low in nutritional value. While such beverages do contribute to weight gain by adding substantially to caloric intake, sodas or beers could further lead to obesity due to their high acid and/or phosphate contents.

An epidemiology study of participants in the Framingham Study found that individuals who consume at least 1 soft drink per day had about a 50% higher prevalence of the metabolic syndrome than those consuming <1 soft drink per day. An interesting note found in this study was that the increased metabolic syndrome risk existed even when the individual consumed diet soft drinks instead of a regular soft drink. A high dietary acid load or a high phosphate load from a dietary source could alter calcium homeostasis. Such alteration in calcium homeostasis would worsen existing hypocalcemia from vitamin D deficiency, and, potentially result in a corresponding inhibition of glucose movement into the cell. This inhibition or the lack of the ability of glucose uptake by the cell is the hallmark of "insulin resistance."

Obesity, therefore, can result from an abnormality in calcium homeostasis that stems from a vitamin D deficiency. In my experience with vitamin D, all my diabetic patients have vitamin D insufficiency or deficiency. For those patients that do not have diabetes, the prevalence of vitamin D insufficiency or deficiency in my patient population is about 90% or more. Vitamin D deficiency plays a role as the causative factor for insulin resistance and diabetes.

About 90% of people diagnosed with Type 2 diabetes are obese. Type 2 diabetes occurs through two known processes: beta-cell dysfunction and insulin resistance. Insulin resistance is the hallmark of patients with Type 2 diabetes and can present up to 12 years before diagnosis. By the time diabetes Type 2 is diagnosed, your pancreas beta cells that produce insulin have declined by an average of 50%. The causal relationship between vitamin D deficiency and insulin resistance stem from the role that vitamin D serves in gene regulation. Vitamin D is thought of as a vitamin, yet by classification it really is a hormone. Unlike other vitamins that are water soluble, vitamin D is a cholesterol molecule. Acting like a fat molecule, vitamin D is unique in its ability to be able to cross the cell membrane into the cell nucleus. Within the cell nucleus, vitamin D is involved in gene regulation through the interaction of the active form of the vitamin, 1, 25-dihydroxyvitamin D3, with Vitamin D receptors (VDRs) within the cell nucleus.

Within the nucleus, the active 1,25-dihydroxyvitamin D3-VDR binds to the retinoid X receptor (RXR), forming the VDR-RXR complex. The regulation of gene transcription is by the interactions of the active vitamin D3 acting on the VDR-RXR complex. The product of this VDR-RXR interaction is a protein involved in the regulation of calcium absorption in the intestine. Thus, the role of vitamin D in cell regulation, specifically its ability to activate the VDR-RXR complex, has a unique and vital role in calcium homeostasis.

The vitamin D Gene Regulation Hypothesis

The role of vitamin D in glucose metabolism or its association with diabetes is unknown. The protein product of the VDR-RXR interaction is a transport protein. Transport proteins facilitate the movement of molecules, such as sugars and amino acids, across the plasma membranes of most cells. I hypothesize that a protein involved in the co-transport of glucose, calcium, and or phosphate across the cell membrane would play an integral part in glucose homeostasis. Moreover, if a condition exists in which the synthesis of this transport proteins is limited, then the appearance of "insulin resistance" would result. A major advancement in the treatment of diabetes was possible when the first thiazolidinedione (TZD), troglitazone, came onto the market in 1997. Troglitazone represented a new oral medication that was effective in not only lowering blood sugar but also possibly slowing down the progression of diabetes itself. Other thiazolidinediones (TZD), rosiglitazone and pioglitzaone soon followed. These three TZDs, classified as peroxisome proliferator-activated receptors (PPARs) agonist, specifically PPAR-gamma agonists, are able to lower blood sugar by increasing insulin sensitivity, primarily through an effect on muscle, liver or adipose tissue. TZDs may also preserve beta cell function.

Interestingly, the PPARs are receptors that exist in the nucleus of a variety of tissues, such as muscle, kidney, fat, liver and macrophages. The PPAR agonists exert their action by the activation and deactivation of genes that regulate glucose and lipid homeostasis and insulin sensitivity. In the nucleus, the PPAR agonist action occurs through the binding with the retinoid X receptor (RXR), which, as previously discussed, is the same receptor to which the activated VDR binds to form the VDR-RXR complex.

Since both the PPAR agonist and the VDR binds to the RXR, it seems reasonable to conclude that agents of the PPAR class must lead to the production of a protein that is dependent on the RXR. In the case of the active vitamin D, a calcium transport protein potentially results. Could the PPAR-RXR interaction result in a similar transport protein, one that is responsible for the transport of glucose, calcium and phosphate from extracellular to intracellular and the transport of sodium in the opposite direction? Sodium is included as an electrolyte associated with this transport protein because of the high frequency of reported edema associated with TZD. This edema, which can lead to congestive heart failure, is the likely result of the transportation of sodium across the cell membrane that is opposite to the movement of calcium, glucose, and phosphate.

If the gene product in the interaction of the PPAR/VDR-RXR complex is indeed a trans-membrane protein involved in the transport of glucose, calcium, phosphate and sodium, then a vitamin D deficiency would explain the mechanism for insulin resistance.

Given the proposed mechanism of vitamin D in cell regulation, insulin resistance could be an effect of 1, 25-dihydroxyvitamin D3 deficiency. The fundamental low level of active vitamin D results in a corresponding decrease in the action of the RXR receptor on gene expression. This, in turn, leads to an absence of or a decrease in the synthesis of the transport protein product, and, therefore, potentially inhibiting glucose movement across the cell membrane. The inability to transport glucose into the cell creates a relative hypoglycemic intracellular and hyperglycemic extracellular state. Normal regulatory processes respond, stimulating the release of insulin from the pancreas to control the "hyperglycemia."

This hypothesis, therefore, points to the initial vitamin D deficiency as the primary cause of an ensuing insulin resistance. Furthermore, the consequent rise in insulin acts to transport glucose into energy storing tissues, such as adipose tissue, and to the liver for lipid synthesis. In this way, the mechanism triggered by vitamin D deficiency leads to hyperlipidemia, as well. The hyperlipidemia resulting from this process could be a consequence of an effort to create an alternative fuel source to spare glucose for the brain and/or the role of cholesterol as a precursor for the synthesis of vitamin D and other hormones, such as cortisol and corticosteroids. Moreover, beta cell failure, the second core defect of Type 2 diabetes, could be a result of beta cell death caused by a lack of calcium, an essential electrolyte.

Poison is in everything, and no thing is without poison. The dosage makes it either a poison or a remedy.

– Philipus Aureolus Paracelsus

Memory and Dementia

As you age, your ability to learn and remember new information seems to get worse. This is what I hear from my older patients, family and friends. The fact is that I do agree that as you age, your memory is not what it was when you are younger. Nevertheless, a person's cognitive ability will vary but for the most part, it should remain relatively stable over his or her lifetime. Some individuals will have declines in memory and processing speed that are noticeable only to others but not severe enough to interfere with daily life. For most, this mild cognitive decline does not progress to dementia. Yet the question is why does your memory or ability to remember and learn information worsen with age?

Some reasons for memory deficit not related to aging are from health conditions such as stroke or other specific diseases that affect brain function. The current wisdom is that memory deficits are common, as you get older and happen more as a rule than an exception. However, aging is not the reason for the inability to remember and learn information as you age. Using age as an explanation is an attempt to explain away something that is not yet understood. Aging does not have to result in memory deficit. Other explanations and factors more critical in maintaining memory are likely the real reason for memory deficit.

Dementia is defined as a progressive deterioration of multiple aspects of cognitive ability, with memory and other functions such as learning, orientation, language, comprehension or judgment, severe enough to interfere with daily life. The National Institute of Neurological Disorder and Stroke defines dementia not as a specific disease but as a descriptive term for a collection of symptoms causing impairment of intellectual function. Individuals with dementia have impairment of normal daily living activities such as problem solving, emotions and personality. They also have behavior problems such as agitation, delusions, and hallucinations. Dementia occurs when "two or more brain functions, such as memory and language skills, are significantly impaired without any loss of consciousness." This diagnostic definition is broader in scale compared to Alzheimer's. The reason for this is that Alzheimer's initially affects short-term memory and then progresses to affect other aspects of daily function.

The most common form of dementia, Alzheimer's, currently affects about 5 million Americans and accounts for an estimated 60% to 80% of all dementia. It is currently the sixth-leading cause of death in the United States. Alzheimer's is a progressive neurodegenerative disease that is characterized by the inability to learn new information (although more recent research has shown that Alzheimer's patients can still learn, although on a smaller scale than normal). Alzheimer's eventually robs affected individuals of their memories, their reasoning abilities, and their personalities.

In the early part of Alzheimer's, distant information or memories are preserved. The initial signs and symptoms of Alzheimer's are individuals with the inability to recall new events or new information. The memory deficit is of short-term memory. As Alzheimer progresses, other areas -- such as the ability to reason, make judgments, and communication -- are affected. In the later stage of Alzheimer, all aspects of daily living are affected. The causes for the "memory loss" as you age are often unknown. However, the reason for the inability to learn or remember new information as you age will not be such a mystery if you look at the lack of proper nutrition as the cause. I believe that most "memory loss" that occurs with aging is due to a slow, insidious process that is uniquely tied to malnutrition.

The lack of an appetite as you age is common. The reason my patients give as to why they are not eating is that they are not hungry or they lack an appetite. The explanation for a lack of appetite as you age is unknown, except to say again that it is believed to be a common normal process of aging. However, I believe a more logical explanation besides aging exists. *As you age, your appetite decreases since your metabolism has been reset secondarily to malnutrition.* The fact is that if you are malnourished, then your metabolic rate will slow down due to the resulting malnutrition. Your body's basal metabolic rate will have to slow down to match the shortage of available nutrients from the foods eaten. Once you are deficient in certain essential nutrients, the consequence of this is that the body tries to conserve the existing nutrients by way of a slower metabolic rate. This will translate to a decreased appetite. With a lower metabolic rate and a decreased appetite, nutritional deficiencies will only worsen the problem. It will result in further adverse health. This explanation illustrates how your body's homeostatic mechanism works in dealing with a real life situation of an inadequate supply causing a slower demand.

Since we do not yet know how our brain works in the way of information storage, I will need to speculate on how you are able to store data. Understanding how your brain stores information is important, since I believe that this process becomes defective in Alzheimer's. The reason for the inability to learn new information is possibly due to the inability to store new information or to recall the new information that was stored. I believe that the key nutrient that plays a role in information storage and thus memory is protein. As mentioned earlier, the amino acids found in proteins are the physical nutrients that your body uses to record and store information. Your body will likely use the amino acids from dietary protein to form new protein structures that will actually be important for memory. If you think about what you are composed of and what the foods you eat are composed of, protein is the nutrient most likely to play a role in information storage. I theorized that, in individuals with Alzheimer's, the macronutrient deficient that predisposes them to it is protein.

I believe that the inability to learn and remember new information, the early signs of Alzheimer, is the results of your brain's inability to store new information as short-term memory. The storage of new information is not possible due to an acute nutritional deficiency on top of an overall existing chronic deficiency of protein and other micronutrients. Keep in mind when I say protein malnutrition or micronutrients deficiency exists, the nutrients that I am referring to may be available but not necessarily in the amounts needed to fulfill your daily demands. The nutrients that are deficient may not be absolute but only a relative deficiency in the amount-needed to serve the function-required at that specific moment.

If your body needs certain amino acids and they are not available, it will not be able to maintain the same number of cells for any organ system. This is also true for your brain. Your brain needs proteins to maintain its size and function. Think of your brain as an organ similar to your muscle. With inadequate protein intake, your muscle will shrink up. This will also happen to your brain. From a building blocks standpoint, the effect of protein malnutrition on your brain is the same as it is on your muscles. With protein malnutrition, your brain's ability to maintain the same number of brain cells you have today as tomorrow and beyond is compromised.

I believe that the reason proteins are important in memory is that memory formation and storage are retained in proteins. The reason why you cannot form short-term memory is due to your brain's inability to store any new information in the form of new proteins. These new proteins should be from the amino acids that are available from your daily dietary protein intake. Eating a diet insufficient for daily protein requirement will not provide your body with the amino acids it needs in order to build new proteins or to repair "old protein." Proteins play a role in both short term and long-term memory. The information stored, as short term or long-term memories are formed from protein. The difference between short term and long-term memory is timing; long-term memory was formed and finalized before short-term memory.

If the initial process of memory formation does not occur, due to an amino acid deficiency, then the ability to form short-term memory will not occur. Memory or informational data not stored, as new proteins will not be recalled as memory since it was never stored as new proteins. From this example, you can see how memory formations are affected by protein malnutrition.

Another nutrient that may be deficient and can cause Alzheimer's is a deficiency of the vitamin B, choline. You need choline to help you create the neurotransmitter acetylcholine. The synthesis of acetylcholine requires choline to be present as it is the choline part of the acetylcholine. A deficiency in choline could affect memory since it would present as a decrease in acetylcholine synthesis and availability. A lowered acetylcholine level is not optimal for your brain's health. Acetylcholine is important in memory function since current medications used for Alzheimer's acts to increase acetylcholine availability.

In Alzheimer's, short-term memories are the first to be affected. Think of short-term memories as information that your visual sensory organs, such as your eyes, records. Imagine that your eyes are like a movie camera that records everything that happens during the span of a day. The information recorded by your eyes will need to be stored and organized. I believe that the storage and organization of our daily events occurs during sleep. Your short-term memories are "recorded" on or as new proteins within your neuronal cells. Think of your neuronal cells as being similar to a computer memory chip. For a computer memory chip, information is stored as an electrical signal with either on or off as 1 or 0. In a similar fashion, your body could use the dietary amino acids to form new protein structures that then act as the 1 and 0 similar to a memory chip's 1 and 0.

Over an extended period, the initial impact of protein malnutrition on brain function will be on short-term memory. The reason for this is that short-term memory formation is uniquely dependent on daily dietary amino acids. Short-term memory formation should not compromise tissue amino acids or proteins that are already being used for other functions. Daily dietary protein is supposed to supply your body with the additional amino acids needed for recent new memory formation. This explanation is the reason why you cannot seem to remember "anything" during stressful times. During such times, it is likely that your dietary intake of proteins and other micronutrients needed for brain function or bodily function is inadequate.

With the continued worsening of daily protein malnutrition, this eventually leads to problems with long-term memory. Long-term memories are also formed from amino acids. However, since long-term memories were formed prior to the protein malnutrition, it is logical that they should be "preserved" and not affected to the same degree as short-term memory. Eventually, long-term memories are affected by the continual worsening protein malnutrition needed for proper brain function.

I believe that the evidence for protein malnutrition as the cause for Alzheimer's is there in the brain. One characterizing hallmark of Alzheimer's is the accumulation of abnormal proteins called amyloid plaques and neurofibrillary tangles. Amyloid plaques are protein fragments normally produced by the body and found between nerve cells (neurons) in the brain. Neurofibrillary tangles are insoluble twisted proteins found within the neuron cells. The tangles are proteins called tau, and are proteins that form part of the microtubule system within the nerve cells. Microtubules are protein that helps transport of possible nutrients from one part of the nerve cell to another part of the cell. The etiology of these amyloid plaques and neurofibrillary tangles and their association with Alzheimer's is unknown. However, the fact that amyloid plaques and neurofibrillary tangles are themselves proteins that are denatured is clinically significant. Denatured proteins represent remnant proteins. Remnant proteins are the by-products of the catabolic processes that your body has worked out in dealing with nutritional deficiencies.

This description for the possible mechanism of Alzheimer's is just an illustration of how nutritional deficiencies of the needed micro and macronutrient will affect health and vitality.

By the time nutritional deficiencies finally affect your memory; other aspects of your health have already been severely compromised. Alzheimer's is just one possible example of what can result from severe protein deficiency and the catabolic processes of homeostasis. Individuals having a CT scan of the head for the evaluation of dementia or for other reasons, often show evidence of an overall decrease in brain volume. The decrease in brain volume is called cerebral atrophy and is believed to occur as part of the normal process of aging (some atrophy is also seen with chronic, heavy alcohol use). The current wisdom is that with aging, your brain volume decreases. In fact, it is believed that brain volume decreases by about 2% per decade. The 2% loss of brain size is again considered normal aging. However, the question to then ask is, "Why should your brain size decrease with age?"

I believe a better explanation exists than aging. Cerebral atrophy is not the normal process of aging but is another effect of catabolism. The real reason for the decrease in brain volume, as seen on CT-scans as cerebral atrophy, is due to a severe and prolonged process of protein malnutrition. The chronic effect of protein malnutrition on brain size or anatomy will be cerebral atrophy.

Protein malnutrition and nutritional deficiencies occur daily in everyone. This is the real fact of life. For as long as humans have walked this earth, micro and macronutrient nutritional deficiencies occur without your recognition and are the underlying reasons for the variability in how each individual age. Without adequate micro and macronutrients, which act as the building blocks for your cells, you cannot expect to maintain the same number of brain cells tomorrow as today. A decrease in brain volume represents neuronal cell deaths. The cause for these neuronal cell deaths is from deficiencies such as proteins, vitamins, minerals, and the essential fatty acids. These nutrients support neuronal cell health and function, so when they are deficit, something has to give.

The diffused macroscopic cerebral atrophy seen in aging does not represent the normal process of the aging brain. In addition, in order for things seen on a macroscopic level, it must mean that on the microscopic level, changes in the neuronal cells' microenvironment must have been prolonged and significant. Some of the cerebral atrophy seen on CT-scans is also apparent in the "normal" appearing individual. The significance of such finding is often brushed off as aging or something incurable and unavoidable. Yet, any degree of cerebral atrophy that you see in a "normal" appearing individual should be a warning sign for nutritional deficiencies. A pending underlying nutritional deficiency, if not corrected, will worsen and progress towards dementia.

Individuals with Alzheimer's can experience symptoms such as changes in their personality and behavior, such as anxiety, suspiciousness, agitation, as well as delusions and hallucinations. These symptoms often occur in the late stage of the disease. Currently, age is the most important risk factor for Alzheimer's disease. Yet as discussed previously, age or aging in itself are not the cause for illnesses and diseases. *Age or aging acts as a time factor for setting different events into motion and for nutritional deficiencies to progress.* The real causes for

Alzheimer's or other human diseases are likely due to nutritional deficiencies of the needed nutrients. Nutrients that are deficient are the essential amino acids and the vitamins and minerals needed for cellular metabolism and function. For instance, if the body does not have the nutritional building blocks it needs to replace, repair or maintain the number of brain cells you have today, how can memory be "created" or maintained for tomorrow?

Today, the only definitive way to diagnose Alzheimer's is after an individual suspected of having Alzheimer's dies. The reason for this is that an Alzheimer diagnosis can be confirmed only by looking for characteristic protein deposits found in the brains of individuals with Alzheimer's. The proteins characteristic of Alzheimer's disease are clumps of proteins called amyloid plaques and bundle of fibers called neurofibrillary tangles. These proteins are so prevalent in a brain autopsy of individuals with Alzheimer's disease that it is even thought to be the "inciting" cause for Alzheimer's.

Currently, researchers are trying to find a "cure" for Alzheimer's. The targets for the treatment of Alzheimer's are toward the amyloid plaques and the neurofibrillary tangles. The treatment hypothesis for Alzheimer's rests on the premise of either trying to prevent the amyloid plaques and neurofibrillary tangles from occurring or trying to decrease the amount once it has occurred. The outcome in this approach is to prevent or delay the progression of Alzheimer's. Similarly, researchers are also trying to find indicators for a person's risk of developing Alzheimer's by trying to identify specific proteins, known as biomarker proteins. Biomarker proteins are used to detect proteins in a person's blood or spinal fluid that would indicate an increase risk for

Alzheimer's. This method, if reliable, should then enable a pre mortem diagnosis of Alzheimer's without having to exam a postmortem brain for these proteins. The fact that there are abundances of amyloid plaques and neurofibrillary tangles in a person with Alzheimer's is the reason I believe proteins play a critical key role in "memory storage."

Once a person has Alzheimer's, the amyloid plaques and neurofibrillary tangle proteins that characterize it can represent protein remnants from prior proteins that were used to store memory or from the unformed proteins due to the amino acid deficiencies. From this description, deficiencies in short-term memories are the result of a memory storing process not occurring to completion. Inadequacy of dietary protein occurring over time will deplete your body of the essential amino acids needed for new protein synthesis needed for the memory function. *In fact, lacking any essential amino acids will cause all protein biosynthesis to come to a halt if the protein synthesized requires the essential amino acids that are missing*.

The second explanation for the amyloid plaques and neurofibrillary tangle proteins seen in Alzheimer's patients are that these proteins are the remnants or the by-product of the catabolism or autophagy processes of existing long-term memory protein. Remember that cell death occurs through three possibilities: cell necrosis, program cell death, and catabolism or autophagy. Faced with a nutritional deficiency, beyond a critical point, your body will use its self-digestion process called autophagy. The process of cellular autophagy is the catabolism needed to salvage the essential amino acids required during time of existing dietary protein intake deficiency. Lacking the essential or non-essential amino acids in your brain will create an unfortunate situation that forces your body to breakdown existing memory stored as proteins. The reason why amyloid plaques and neurofibrillary tangle proteins exist is that these proteins are the residual proteins left from the autophagy process. These proteins are the remnant of a once existing memory structure laid previously as protein structures for long-term memory.

Currently there is no cure for Alzheimer's disease because at present we do not understand what causes it. I have presented what I believe are possible causes for Alzheimer's disease: proteins and micronutrients deficiencies such as choline, which are nutrients found in the foods we eat. Thus, I believe that if we become deficient in these two specific nutrients, then we will be predisposed to have a greater chance of getting Alzheimer's disease. Other micro and macronutrients can also play a role in Alzheimer's development but to a lesser extent than protein and choline. If these are the causes for Alzheimer's, then the possible solution is to optimize nutrition in the needed essential nutrients of proteins, vitamins and minerals to "cure" Alzheimer's.

The current medical treatment for Alzheimer's focuses on giving medications that work on increasing the neurotransmitter called acetylcholine. Henry Hallett Dale first identified this neurotransmitter in 1914. Acetylcholine is in both the peripheral nervous system and the central nervous system. Acetylcholine works by binding to acetylcholine receptors and opening sodium channels on different tissue membranes. Acetylcholine receptors are in different locations throughout your body such as the skeletal muscle, cardiac muscle and in the brain, as part of the autonomic nervous system. Acetylcholine effects can be either excitatory or inhibitor depending on where its action is in the body. In skeletal muscles, acetylcholine causes muscle contraction. While in cardiac muscles, it decreases muscle contraction. In the brain and in the parasympathetic part of the autonomic nervous system, acetylcholine effects are stimulatory.

Since there are no current known causes for Alzheimer's, medications are the only approach used to treat the memory deficit in Alzheimer's. Medications that treat Alzheimer's specifically block the enzyme that breakdowns acetylcholine. Therefore, the available acetylcholine is then at a relatively higher level then normally exists. Acetylcholine is an important neurotransmitter in the regulation of memory. How acetylcholine works for memory formation is still unknown. However, as we currently know, using medications that block its breakdown increases the brain's acetylcholine level. From this, I would then presume that acetylcholine must be an important neurotransmitter in the memory process. The effectiveness of medications used for Alzheimer's is minimally effective by the time they are used. Improving nutritional deficiencies might not reverse dementia but the unknown is, "Can further deterioration be slowed or prevented?"

Parkinson's Disease

Parkinson's disease is a neurodegenerative disorder that belongs to a group of conditions known as movement disorders. Thus, the main feature seen in individuals with Parkinson's disease is disorder of movement. Parkinsonism is a term that refers to the syndrome of tremor, rigidity, bradykinesia (abnormal slowness of movement) and postural instability. Parkinson's disease affects both an individual's motor skills and later on their cognition and speech, is the most common cause of Parkinsonism.

The features of Parkinson's disease are due to a decrease in dopamine synthesis within your brain. Dopamine, a neurotransmitter, is synthesis from dopaminergic neurons of the basal ganglia, specifically the substantia nigra. It is believed that with the decrease in dopamine synthesis from the substantia nigra, the amount of dopamine available is not enough to stimulate the region of the motor cortex, thus affecting motor functions.

During my efforts to understand the function and synthesis of dopamine, I discovered the importance and implication of nutrition. Somehow, it never occurred to me to ask the question as to where dopamine comes from. You might wonder what the connection between dopamine and nutrition could be. Actually, it is quite straightforward. I discovered that dopamine is synthesized from tyrosine! By this, I mean tyrosine is the precursor molecule that your body uses to synthesize dopamine. The fact that tyrosine is an amino acid, specifically a non-essential amino acid found in food, became the spark that lit my desire to further understand nutrition.

Tyrosine is an amino acid found only in protein-based foods. It is a nonessential yet "conditional" amino acid due to the availability and demand for it as a precursor. Tyrosine is nonessential because our body can synthesize it endogenously if it has the essential amino acid phenylalanine. If your diet becomes deficient in phenylalanine, then tyrosine becomes an essential amino acid. Tyrosine is a conditional amino acid because there are situations where the body's demand of tyrosine could outstrip its availability. When this happens, then a "relative" deficiency of needed tyrosine arises. I found the fact that your body uses tyrosine for the synthesis of dopamine amazing and revealing, since it made eating protein-based foods that much more important.

Once I discovered the connection between tyrosine and dopamine, I felt that the cause for Parkinson's disease lies in nutrition, or specifically tyrosine and total daily protein deficiency. Parkinson's disease is due to a decrease in dopamine synthesis from neurons of the substantia nigra and secondarily from a decrease in the precursor needed for dopamine synthesis, tyrosine. Increase your brain's tyrosine availability by increasing dietary tyrosine and protein from your diet then more dopamine would be synthesized. The discovery that your body uses proteins or, more specifically, the amino acids from the protein foods was a revelation. Your body synthesizes dopamine through the conversion of tyrosine with the aid of two enzymes, tyrosine hydroxylase and dopamine decarboxylase.

Realizing dopamine is from tyrosine and tyrosine is just one of the twenty amino acids found in protein meant that if we do not consume foods with sufficient tyrosine, the synthesis of dopamine would be limited. Similarly, when other essential amino acids are limited, then your body would be unable to synthesize all the "non-essential" amino acids needed for health.

Tyrosine is a unique amino acid in the sense that it has diverse uses as precursors for multiple neurotransmitters along with thyroid and skin pigmentation functions. Your body's demand for tyrosine is variable compared to other amino acids. Tyrosine insufficiency can occur when the demand for it exceeds its availability. Your body uses tyrosine as a precursor for not only dopamine but also other neurotransmitters such as epinephrine, and norepinephrine.

Tyrosine is also the precursor for melanin and thyroid hormone. An interesting aside: The consequence of tyrosine deficiency shows up as the graying of one's hair color! I know this to be true because I have witnessed it. Of my patients, friends and family members who took tyrosine as directed, all reported that the gray hairs they used to have are slowly disappearing. Since the color of hair is observable and the fact that gray hairs are reversible can be interpreted only one way. *Gray hair is not determined genetically by age but is nutritionally dependent.* The amount of tyrosine taken and the speed in which your gray hair is reversed are dependent on how long you have been graying. The greater amount of gray hair that you have and the longer the duration, the greater dose of tyrosine a person has to take daily in order to begin the reversal process of graying. The aging process does not have to result in gray hair as we currently think it does. If the explanation for a person's gray hair is aging, then giving tyrosine should not reverse their gray hair. However, tyrosine does work in reversing the graying process. Thus, graying cannot be the result of aging, and what is believed to be true about the aging process is probably incorrect.

The reason giving tyrosine works in reversing gray hair is that tyrosine is the precursor to melanin. When you are giving your body the nutrient needed for hair pigmentation, melanin, your hair color will not be gray. This is the only reason why tyrosine works! Many of the illnesses we have are the result of nutritional deficiencies, and if not recognized, will worsen with time. In the aging process, graying occurs due to a deficiency of the precursors for melanin. Tyrosine is a conditional nonessential amino acid, which -- if our body does not have enough of it -- will result in potential deficiencies in melanin, thyroid hormone, dopamine, norepinephrine, and epinephrine.

The discovery that the precursors to a number of vital hormone and neurotransmitters are from protein was the key to my initial understanding of nutrition. Now, I finally understood how an improper diet, specifically the lack of adequate proteins, could affect your health. Staying healthy and vital through the mantra "you are what you eat" is now possible through a proper diet pattern that supplies adequate micro and macronutrients.

The current treatment for Parkinson is based on augmenting the brain's dopamine level by either giving dopamine or by inhibiting the breakdown of dopamine within the neuron. These approaches to the management of Parkinson's disease are effective. However, in most individuals with Parkinson's disease, this treatment only works for a while. Over time, most individuals with Parkinson's disease will worsen regardless of the medications used. I believe that the reason as to why most individuals with Parkinson's disease fail on medications is that the medications do not address the real cause for Parkinson's disease: severe protein malnutrition and tyrosine insufficiency. I believe Parkinson's disease is due to a deficiency of total body proteins needed to maintain dopaminergic neurons function along with an insufficiency of the precursor (the amino acid – tyrosine) needed for dopamine synthesis. Protein malnutrition will decrease the number of dopamine synthesizing neurons as evidenced by the decrease in dopaminergic neurons of the basal ganglia, specifically the substantia nigra. Evidence for neuron cell mass loss is cerebral atrophy.

The fact that tyrosine is the amino acid that your body uses to make dopamine and other important hormone and neurotransmitters was an eye opener for the following reason. If your body does not have enough tyrosine, then you can suffer from not only Parkinson's disease but also hypothyroidism and melanin disorder. The most obvious visible melanin disorder is vitiligo disorder and the graying of one's hair. Hypothyroidism and the graying of your hair are due to a tyrosine insufficiency or deficiency. A tyrosine deficiency can present as a supply and demand problem if tyrosine's availability becomes insufficient for the production of dopamine, thyroid hormone, melanin, norepinephrine, and epinephrine. Graying is reversible with tyrosine supplementation. This is possible regardless of the age of the individual. I have patients that can testified that tyrosine does indeed reverse their gray hair. I have also been able to decrease medication usage for patients with hypothyroidism with tyrosine supplementation.

If detected early enough, Parkinsonism or Parkinson's disease is likely reversible. I believe Parkinsonism or Parkinson's disease is reversible if the protein malnutrition and specifically a tyrosine deficiency are addressed early enough before significant neuronal cell death has occurred. Reversing protein malnutrition could possibly slow the depletion of dopaminergic neurons. Reversing tyrosine insufficiency will increase the precursor for dopamine and possibly force an increase in production of dopamine from those neurons left to produce dopamine. The connection between nutrition and human diseases is that a diet deficient of essential micro and macronutrients will cause the lack of production of enzymes, hormones and neurotransmitters needed for health.

Tyrosine's Importance

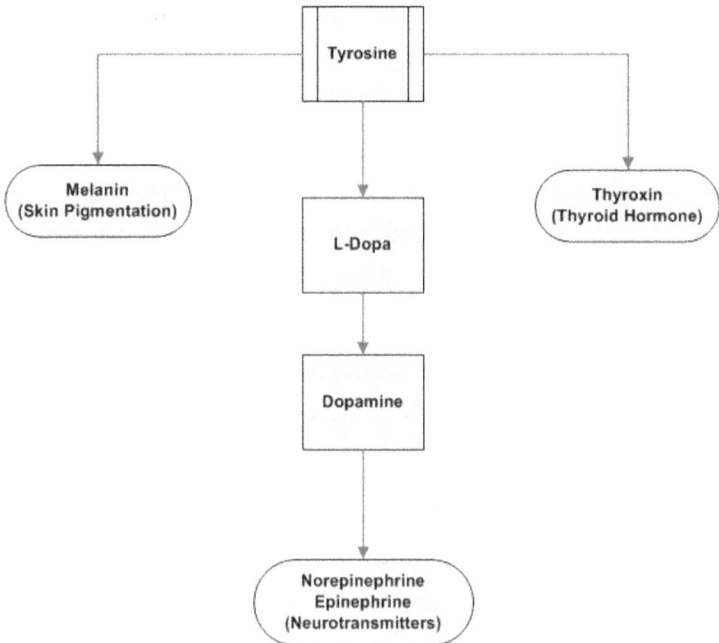

```
                            ┌─────────────┐
              ┌─────────────│  Tyrosine   │──────────────┐
              │             └──────┬──────┘              │
              ▼                    ▼                      ▼
      ┌───────────────┐     ┌─────────────┐      ┌───────────────┐
      │    Melanin    │     │   L-Dopa    │      │   Thyroxin    │
      │(Skin Pigment.)│     └──────┬──────┘      │(Thyroid Horm.)│
      └───────────────┘            │             └───────────────┘
                                   ▼
                            ┌─────────────┐
                            │  Dopamine   │
                            └──────┬──────┘
                                   │
                                   ▼
                          ┌─────────────────┐
                          │  Norepinephrine │
                          │   Epinephrine   │
                          │(Neurotransmit.) │
                          └─────────────────┘
```

Mood Disorders

A common theme discussed so far is that illnesses and diseases are due to imbalances or out right deficiencies of micro and macronutrients. Nutritional imbalances or deficiencies will give rise to signs and symptoms that are then diagnosed as an illness or a disease. *Think about it, your body has no other way to communicate to you that an imbalance or deficiencies in micro and macronutrients exist, except by signs and symptoms.* Treating signs and symptoms will improve it but will not "heal" you. Prescription medication used to treat medical diagnoses will not reverse nutritional imbalances or deficiencies.

Diagnoses such as cardiovascular diseases, cancers, Alzheimer's disease, and Parkinson's disease are all rooted in an underlining nutritional imbalances or deficiencies. Another group of diagnoses also caused by imbalances or deficiencies of nutrients are mood disorders. Genetic susceptibility does play a role in mood disorder. However, nutritional influence is as great or greater than genetic. The clinical manifestation of the severity of an individual's mood disorder is tied to nutrition.

Environmentally, the nutrient most influential in mood disorder is the amino acid L-tryptophan. L-tryptophan is an essential amino acid because your body cannot endogenously synthesize L-tryptophan. The only way you can obtain this essential amino acid is by eating foods that are protein-based and have L-tryptophan as one of the amino acids within them. However, even when you eat foods that are protein based, the amount of L-tryptophan available is usually low.

L-tryptophan is an important amino acid in mood disorder since it is the precursor for serotonin. Serotonin is an important neurotransmitter implicated in mood disorders. The significance of serotonin and mood disorders is unknown. Yet, it seems that the medication used to treat mood disorder seems to work by raising individuals' serotonin level in their brain and this improves mood. L-tryptophan is also the precursor for niacin and melatonin. Melatonin is an important chemical needed for sleep regulation.

L-tryptophan Metabolism

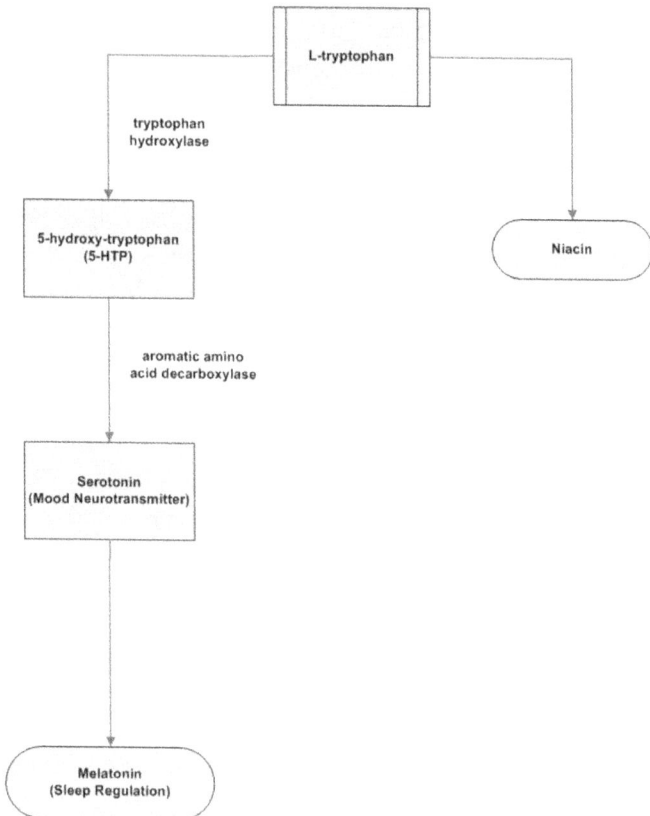

Serotonin is an important neurotransmitter in the regulation of emotions. Your body makes serotonin from L-tryptophan. Understanding L-tryptophan metabolism and function will be helpful in understanding mood disorders, which was my interest. I wanted to understand how medications used to treat mood disorders work. I also wanted to know the factors important in determining which medications would or would not be effective in different individuals. For instance, the commonly used prescription medications used for depression, anxiety, phobia, or obsessive-compulsive disorder are a group of medications known as selective serotonin reuptake inhibitors (SSRI). SSRIs work by selectively inhibiting postsynaptic site neuronal cells from reuptake of serotonin. The SSRI mechanism of action is to increase serotonin level by inhibiting its breakdown and reuptake back into the postsynaptic nerve cell. SSRI also work to increase other neurotransmitters such as dopamine and norepinephrine levels by inhibiting their degradation.

To understand how serotonin might work, the question to consider is, does a low serotonin level within the post-synaptic sites cause mood disorders? The assumption would be yes, since medications that increase serotonin levels at the post-synaptic sites seem to improve an individual's mood. Answering this question would then lead you to believe that symptoms of mood disorders is improved, if and only if the low states of serotonin activity at post-synaptic sites are responsible for the abnormal mood seen in mood disorders.

SSRIs works by increasing the neurotransmitter levels at postsynaptic receptors site by inhibiting their breakdowns. Since this is the case, the next question to ask is, "Why are some individuals' post-synaptic serotonin levels low to begin with?" The question to explain this would be, "Why serotonin levels are low at the postsynaptic receptor sites?" To explain why serotonin levels are low in individuals with mood disorders, you should start by looking at how your body makes serotonin. Your body synthesizes serotonin from L-tryptophan, an essential amino acid. Essential amino acids are not synthesized endogenously within your body. The only way you will obtain them is to consume protein-based foods daily. Moreover, as before, protein deficiencies will limit the amount of essential and non-essential amino acids your body has to work with -- in the case of mood disorder, L-tryptophan for serotonin and tyrosine for dopamine and norepinephrine.

Protein deficiency is common and occurs due to a dietary imbalance of the macronutrients consumed. A diet with too many carbohydrates and not enough proteins, as required for your body weight and metabolism, predisposes you to a greater chance of mood disorders. For individuals who consume too many carbohydrates or have a sweet tooth, they know that eating carbohydrates are addicting. How I explain this addiction to carbohydrates is: Eating too many carbohydrates, which means your body has less of the L-tryptophan available to synthesize to serotonin; less serotonin, in turn, means less will power to stop eating carbohydrates and more carbohydrate cravings leading to increased chances for mood disorders. The second explanation is that when you do not give your body what it needs in the form of micro or macronutrients, your body will sense these as deficiencies, cause continual hunger, and drive you to eat. The problem with this cycle is that the foods that you are eating will not fulfill those nutritional deficiencies and thus the signal for hunger continues.

In discussing the treatment of mood disorders, the neurotransmitters thought to play an important role in causing mood disorder are imbalances of serotonin, dopamine, and norepinephrine. Serotonin is the main neurotransmitter that all SSRIs work on. Antidepressant medications work by increasing the serotonin levels in your brain at sites where nerve communication is occurring. This effect seems to make a person with mood disorder feel better.

It was not until I understood that serotonin came from the essential amino acid L-tryptophan that I finally figured out the fact that a person with a mood disorder might have insufficient precursor amounts of L-tryptophan needed for serotonin synthesis. From this point of view, depression and other mood disorders, where serotonin is involved, are due to a shortage of the precursor amino acid needed for synthesis of serotonin, dopamine and norepinephrine. Your body's capacity to synthesize serotonin is dependent on the amount of L-tryptophan available. The amount is dependent on our dietary intake of L-tryptophan. An inadequate amount of L-tryptophan will limit our body's capacity to convert L-tryptophan to serotonin; an inadequate amount of tyrosine causes dopamine and norepinephrine insufficient or deficiency. Both of these neurotransmitters are associated with mood disorders.

A factor as important as having the needed precursor amino acids is having the enzymes required to convert L-tryptophan into serotonin. The two enzymes required for serotonin synthesis are L-tryptophan hydroxylase and aromatic amino acid decarboxylase. These enzymes are used to convert L-tryptophan into serotonin. Without these enzymes functioning properly, mood disorder can result. Factors that affect the availability of these two enzymes are either nutritional or genetic. In fact, from a genetic standpoint, if a person has a defect in either one or both of the enzymes, they will probably have a greater chance of manifesting a mood disorder. The enzymatic activity level of these two enzymes will determine how well L-tryptophan converts into serotonin. *The activity level of these two enzymes accounts for the genetic inheritability of mood disorder.*

To illustrate this point, let's say that L-tryptophan is A and serotonin is B. L-tryptophan (A) is the precursor and serotonin (B) is the product. The primary factor determining how much of B is synthesized, is by L-tryptophan availability. The second factor that determines how much of B is formed is the activity of the two enzymes, L-tryptophan hydroxylase and aromatic amino acid decarboxylase. These two enzymes are the enzymes that actually convert A to B. How efficiently the two enzymes function is first genetically determined, and second nutritionally dependent. Mood disorders tend to have a genetic prevalence. This prevalence can be explained due to the variability in how well these two enzymes work in converting L-tryptophan into serotonin.

From a genetic standpoint, if an individual has decreased ability to synthesize serotonin due to a lowered activity in L-tryptophan hydroxylase or aromatic amino acid decarboxylase activity, then the synthesis of serotonin is decreased. The decreased enzymatic activity due to a genetic variant in how these two enzymes are coded, along with an environmentally induced nutritional deficiency, will increase the risk of a serotonin deficiency. If serotonin deficiency indeed causes mood disorder, then the connection between how genetic and environmental factors can predispose an individual or a family line to have mood disorder is now evident.

What Does the Evidence Show?

I have come to believe that when you are looking for evidences to back up what you believe is fact; there will be other studies that contradict your belief. This is how it is in the current world we live in. The difference between majorities versus a minority is one percentage point. This conclusion is something I am beginning to accept, as I am uncertain how the information presented in this book will be accepted. What I would ask of my reader is one thing. Think critically.

When you examine different studies regarding nutrition and its effects on health, the results are mixed, inconclusive or confusing. Some studies will show positive results with one supplement but not others. Similarly, for every positive result, you will find a negative one. Why is there such confusion regarding the health benefits with nutritional supplementation or what I really think should be proper nutrition? One reason is because studies that look at nutrition only look at the vitamins and minerals component. What is not yet recognized is that optimal heath is about getting all the parts of nutrition right and not just one part of it.

One vitamin, one mineral or a combination of vitamins or mineral along with any specific eating pattern will not show repeatable positive outcome if other crucial parts are missing. Besides the micronutrients of vitamins and minerals, there are also the macronutrients such as proteins and the essential fatty acids that one can be deficient in that would then lead to poor outcomes. Most studies will test either single micronutrient or a combination of them and not look at optimal nutrition by looking at both micro and macronutrients. No single micronutrient will work in everyone because other nutrients critical to health could be missed. Studies looking individually at vitamins, antioxidants, or proteins will not have consistent positive results because this is not optimal nutrition. There are always nutrients that can be missed and if not corrected, will affect overall health.

Other reasons as to why confusion exists about the health benefits regarding nutrition is that studies are biased toward certain beliefs. People's actions are influenced toward personal, financial, or political gains. As such, the information that you receive and learn in certain aspects may be tainted, unknown to you, toward these biased views. Since writing this book, I have come to view all information that I receive more critically. Two questions I ask myself when judging information: Is the information I am hearing or learning really a fact or is it someone's truth? The difference between a fact and someone else's truth is important. Take time to think for yourself or try to find the answers yourself.

As I have stressed throughout this book, the importance of protein as a vital nutrient needed for health is not recognized. This can be seen clearly in the Dietary Guidelines for Americans 2005, a joint project by the Department of Health and Human Services and Department of Agriculture. This guideline is "the federal government's science-based advice to promote health and reduce risk of chronic diseases through nutrition and physical activity." Within this guideline, 23 of 41 key recommendations are directed toward the public. The rest of the 18 recommendation were for "special populations." The 23 key recommendations are grouped into nine general topics; adequate nutrients within calorie needs, weight management, physical activity, food groups to encourage, fats, carbohydrates, sodium and potassium, alcoholic beverages, and food safety. *The importance of protein as a vital nutrient and its role in health is not even mentioned in any of these 23 recommendations.*

Studies looking at protein supplements do not seem to show that it can enhance athletic performance. Yet most athletes will consume a diet with a higher than usual protein requirement than is expected for most of us -- which now lies at about 10-15% of total daily caloric intake. The lack of direct correlation between protein supplementation and performances is due to other factors beyond the intended effects of protein supplement. Protein supplementation is to provide your body with an optimal amount of essential and non-essential amino acids so it can form other essential proteins needed for bodily function. Protein supplementation cannot enhance performance potential if there are also other components of nutrition that are deficient.

A study by researchers at the University of California San Diego looking at any potential benefit in the supplementation of folic acid and vitamin B for mild to moderate Alzheimer's did not show any slowing in the cognitive decline in Alzheimer's patients. The B vitamins used are the vitamin b12 and vitamin b6. Remember my earlier discussion regarding choline as a B vitamin. This vitamin was not part of the B vitamins used in the study. Choline is an important B vitamin that plays a role as part of the neurotransmitter acetylcholine, which drug therapy for Alzheimer's works on. Similarly, even if the B vitamin choline was of a sufficient amount, a deficiency in protein could still be the overriding cause behind Alzheimer's and not just choline.

Factors to consider in optimal nutrition are that the nutrients needed for bodily function need optimizing and any single nutrient deficieny is not optimal. It is important to have all micro and macronutrients available in adequate amount in order to have optimal health and vigor. The lack of recognition of the prevalence of vitamin D deficiency and its health effects account for an untold amount of preventable medical illnesses and diseases. *In fact, I believe that if everyone on this earth had their vitamin D level checked and those that are deficient get it corrected, then most of the diseases that vitamin D has been linked with would simply disappear.*

Nothing in the world is more dangerous than sincere ignorance and conscientious stupidity.

– Martin Luther King, Jr.

Conclusion

My hope for writing this book is that you can benefit from what I know. The information presented is my way of telling you how you can find the path towards health and vitality. The answers to causes for medical illnesses and diseases are there if you know where to look. I have tried to put together bit and pieces of information from a wide source of disciplines together like pieces of a jigsaw puzzle. Some of the topics discussed in this book, of course, are just theories and concepts and need further investigation. In some ways, certain theories lead to answers that seem too simplistic to be true.

The thing that I believe most of all is that the answers to those topics discussed just seem to make sense. Logically, the answers seem to explain things so easily and in some ways too obviously. The real secret in being able to understand something is to start from the foundation as the first level and work upwards. Going back to the basics gave me a chance to rationalize and explain some unknowns. Information as medical dogma needs to be re-examined. I hope I have given more answers than those that currently exist. The information I presented as hypotheses, to use an analogy, can be considered as looking at things from the forest standpoint of view instead of the trees. To paraphrase an adage that is true, "the devil is in the details." However, this is where the scientific methods will be able to weed out fact versus speculation.

A question I have often asked myself is "Why write a book about my thoughts and theories?" The answer to this question lies in the title of this book, "To know and tell." To know and tell is my way of expressing what I know. To communicate that information so that others may possibly benefit from this information is my goal. I feel that the information presented here can benefit others as it has benefited my family, my patients and me. Another reason I felt the need and desire to tell is that I believe knowing something is not enough. To know something that can improve health and not share it is not to know.

I know that by expressing my views and theories, I may be wrong. To be in error I can accept. I know that there will be skeptics and critics of my writing. I am not afraid to be wrong. To be wrong will give me a chance to correct my mistakes and refine my hypotheses. I will accept that my writing may be incorrect if new facts change my theories.

What I am afraid of is to be right and not to have shared this knowledge. I want to say one day, "Yes, father, you helped me find my way to cure not only Parkinson's disease, but improve health." On that day, I want to be able to say, "It is my dad that you have to thank."

The art of healing comes from nature, not from the physician. Therefore, the physician must start from nature, with an open mind.

– Philipus Aureolus Paracelsus

The grand aim of all science is to cover
The greatest number of empirical facts by logical
deduction
From the smallest number of hypotheses or axioms.

– Albert Einstein

Cowardice asks the question, 'Is it safe?' Expediency asks the question, 'Is it politic?' Vanity asks the question, 'Is it popular?' But, conscience asks the question, 'Is it right?' And there comes a time when one must take a position that is neither safe, nor politic, nor popular, but one must take it because one's conscience tells one that it is right.

– Martin Luther King, Jr.

How to Revise the Nutritional Guidelines

Do not think of nutrition in terms of food groups and amount of servings needed per day.

Think of nutrition in terms of micronutrient (eg. vitamins, minerals) and macronutrients (eg. carbohydrates, proteins, and fats) and the needed amounts in term of body weight

Change the total daily calories intake for macronutrients from:

Carbohydrate 60% + Protein 10% + Lipid 30%

TO

Carbohydrate ≤ 30% + Protein ≥ 35% + Lipid 35%

Carbohydrate needed per day is equal to ≤ 0.75 gram of carbohydrate per 1 pound of body weight

Protein needed per day is equal to ≥ 0.875 gram of protein per 1 pound of body weight.

Fat needed per day is equal to 0.385 gram of fat per 1 pound of body weight. Concentrate on the essential fatty acid such as the EPA/DHA omega -3 fatty acid, supplement with at least 2 to 3 grams a day.

Incorporating the Concepts
Discussed

1) Calculate the number of grams of protein needed per day. Consider daily protein intake anywhere from 35% to 40% (0.87 to 1 gram per pound of body weight).

2) Calculate the total macronutrient calories needed per day. (Body weight in pounds times 10 Kcal/pounds = metabolic rate at rest)

3) Divide total protein calories needed per day by three. Suggestion:

   "Eat breakfast like a king, lunch like a prince, and dinner like a pauper." – Adelle Davis

4) Eat the total grams of protein required per day in divided meals daily. Eat the protein first, then fruits and vegetables afterwards. Avoid "starchy" fruits and vegetables.

5) For carbohydrates keep total carbohydrate intake less then 30 % of total daily caloric intake or less than 0.75 gram per pound.

6) Avoid refine process food sources, limit added sweeteners: high fructose corn syrup. Eat low glycemic index carbohydrate.

7) Supplement daily with added: multi-vitamins, Vitamin B-complex, Vitamin C, Vitamin D, essential fatty acids (EFA), and others.

Appendix

Current FDA Nutritional Guidelines

They are based on the food pyramid, which has just been replaced by MyPlate (which uses a meal plate as an icon rather than a pyramid).

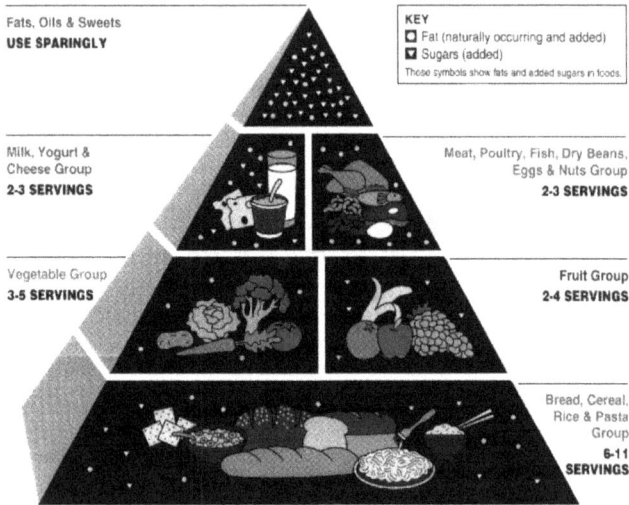

http://en.wikipedia.org/wiki/Food_guide_pyramid

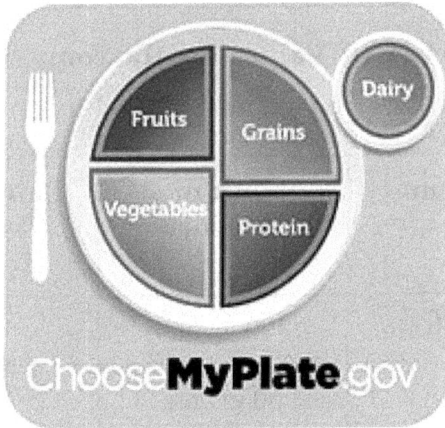

http://en.wikipedia.org/wiki/MyPlate

The food pyramid (MyPlate) broken down into percentages of macronutrients are distributed as USDA Daily Values.

Total daily calories as a % = Carbohydrate 60% + Protein 10%+ Fats 30%

(CPF ratio 60/10/30)

*Calculation for protein requirement based on
the USDA Daily Values versus RDA versus Ideal*

USDA Daily Values for Macronutrients

(Based on a 2000 Calorie Intake)

Nutrient	Unit of Measure	Daily Values (% of daily calories)
Carbohydrate	300 grams	60%
Protein	50 grams	10%
Total Fat	67 grams	30%

Energy requirement:

100 kg person x 20 kcal/kg/day = 2000 kcal/day

Carbohydrate:

60% x 2000 kcal/day = 1200 kcal/day

1200 kcal/day ÷ 4 kcal/gram = 300 grams/day

Protein:

10% x 2000 kcal/day = 200 kcal/day

200 kcal/day ÷ 4 kcal/gram = 50 grams/day

Fat:

30% x 2000 kcal/day = 600 kcal/day

600 kcal/day ÷ 9 kcal/gram = 67 grams/day

Actual Value Based on the RDA

(Based on a 2000 Calorie Intake)

Nutrient	Unit of Measure	Daily Values (% of daily calories)
Carbohydrate	270 grams	54%
Protein	80 grams	16%
Total Fat	67 grams	30%

Current RDA for protein is 0.8 gram/ kilogram/ day

There are 2.2 lbs per 1 kilogram:

(0.8 gram/kilogram)(1 Kilogram) = (x gram) (2.2 lbs)

x = 0.36 gram per 1 lbs

Energy requirement:

100 kg x 20 kcal/kg/day = 2000 kcal/day

Carbohydrate:

54% x 2000 kcal/day = 1080 kcal/day

1080 kcal/day ÷ 4 kcal/gram = 270 grams/day

Protein:

16% x 2000 kcal/day = 320 kcal/day

320 kcal/day ÷ 4 kcal/gram = 80 grams/day

Fat:

30% x 2000 kcal/day = 600 kcal/day

600 kcal/day ÷ 9 kcal/gram = 67 grams/day

USDA Daily Value of 10 % daily protein is suboptimal.

RDA 16% daily protein is better but should be considered the minimal amount needed to maintain lean muscle mass.

AMDR allows the percentage of daily protein to range from 10% to 35%.

Ideal Value Based on the Maximal AMDR
Allowable Protein / Fat Distribution

(Based on a 2000 Calorie Intake)

Nutrient	Unit of Measure	Daily Values (% of daily calories)
Carbohydrate	150 grams	30%
Protein	175 grams	35%
Total Fat	78 grams	35%

Energy requirement:

100 kg person x 20 kcal/kg/day = 2000 kcal/day

Carbohydrate:

30% x 2000 kcal/day = 600 kcal/day

600 kcal/day ÷ 4 kcal/gram = 150 grams/day

Protein:

35% x 2000 kcal/day = 700 kcal/day

700 kcal/day ÷ 4 kcal/gram = 175 grams/day

Fat:

35% x 2000 kcal/day = 700 kcal/day

700 kcal/day ÷ 9 kcal/gram = 78 grams/day

Theoretical Ideal percentage of Protein Distribution

(Based on a 2000 Calorie Intake)

Nutrient	Unit of Measure	Daily Values (% of daily calories)
Carbohydrate	150 grams	30%
Protein	200 grams	40%
Total Fat	67 grams	30%

Energy requirement:

100 kg person x 20 kcal/kg/day = 2000 kcal/day

Carbohydrate:

30% x 2000 kcal/day = 600 kcal/day

600 kcal/day ÷ 4 kcal/gram = 150 grams/day

Protein:

40% x 2000 kcal/day = 800 kcal/day

800 kcal/day ÷ 4 kcal/gram = 200 grams/day

Fat:

30% x 2000 kcal/day = 600 kcal/day

600 kcal/day ÷ 9 kcal/gram = 67 grams/day

The theoretical 200 grams of protein a day for a 100 kg person is 2 grams of protein per 1 kilogram. This is also equivalent to about 1 gram of protein per 1 pound of body weight.

Theoretical Ideal percentage of Protein Distribution

Nutrient	Weight		Daily Values (% of daily calories)
	kg	lb	
Carbohydrate	150 grams	75 grams	30%
Protein	**200 grams**	**100 grams**	**40%**
Total Fat	67 grams	33.5 grams	30%

Note: 1 kg = 2.2 lbs (we will round down to 2)

Energy requirement:

100 kg person x 20 kcal/kg/day = 2000 kcal/day

100 lb person x 10 kcal/kg/day = 1000 kcal/day

References

Preface

The Livin' La Vida Low – Carb Show with Jimmy Moore

Dyer, Wayne: *Inspiration – Your Ultimate Calling*, 2001. Audio book

Gladwell, Malcolm. *Outliers: The Story of Success.* Prod. and Dir. John McElroy. Hachette Audio, 2008. Audio book.

You Are What You Eat

Flegal, K. M., Carroll, M. D., & Ogden, C. L. (2010). Prevalence and Trends in Obesity Among US Adults, 1999-2008. *JAMA.* 303(3), 235–241.

How Do I Know?

Jacob AN, Pho LQ, Jacob KN, A Case of Newly Diagnosed Type 2 Diabetes and Vitamin D Deficiency, *Endocrine Society's Annual Meeting- Endo 2009.*

Wurtman, R. J., Hefti, F., & Melamed, E. (1980). Precursor Control of Neurotransmitter Synthesis. *Pharmacological Reviews*, 32(4), 315–335.

Nutrition

Dietary Reference Intakes for Energy, Carbohydrate, Fiber, Fat, Fatty Acids, Cholesterol, Protein, and Amino Acids (Macronutrients). (2005). *National Academy of Sciences*, 769-879.

Fundamentals of Nutrition. UCLA Center for Human Nutrition.<http://www.cellinteractive.com/ucla/physcia n_ed/fund_nut.html#> [Reviewed 07 July 2011].

Carbohydrates

Dietary Reference Intakes for Energy, Carbohydrate, Fiber, Fat, Fatty Acids, Cholesterol, Protein, and Amino Acids (Macronutrients). (2005). *National Academy of Sciences*, 769-879.

Proteins

Fundamentals of Human Nutrition. <www.cellinteractive.com/ucla/physcian_ed/fund_nut.h tml > [Reviewed 07 July 2011].

Harper, A. E., & Yoshimura, N. N. (September/October 1993). Amino Acid Balance -- Full Technical Report on Amino Acid Balance and Usage in the Body. <http://www.oralchelation.com/technical/amino1.htm# 14> [Reviewed 07 July 2011].

Martin WF, Armstrong LE, Rodriguez NR. Dietary protein intake and renal function. *Nutr Metab* (Lond). 2005 Sep 20;2:25.

Otten, J. J., Hellwig, J. P., & Meyers, L. D. (2006). *Dietary Reference Intakes: The Essential Guide to Nutrient Requirements*, 144-155.

Phenylketonuria: MedlinePlus Medical Encyclopedia. (2009). National Institutes of Health. <http://www.nlm.nih.gov/medlineplus/ency/article/001166.htm> [Reviewed 07 July 2011].

Report of Joint WHO FAO UNU Expert Consultation (2007). Protein and Amino Acid Requirements in Human Nutrition. <http://whqlibdoc.who.int/trs/WHO_TRS_935_eng.pdf> [Reviewed 07 July 2011].

Symons TB, Sheffield-Moore M, Wolfe RR, Paddon-Jones D. A moderate serving of high-quality protein maximally stimulates skeletal muscle protein synthesis in young and elderly subjects. *J Am Diet Assoc*. 2009 Sep;109(9):1582-6.

Westerterp-Plantenga MS. Protein intake and energy balance. *Regul Pept*. 2008 Aug 7;149(1-3):67-9.

Lipids

Dietary Reference Intakes for Energy, Carbohydrate, Fiber, Fat, Fatty Acids, Cholesterol, Protein, and Amino Acids (Macronutrients) (2005). *National Academy of Sciences*, 769-879.

Liu S, Willett WC, Stampfer MJ, Hu FB, Franz M, Sampson L, Hennekens CH, Manson JE. A prospective study of dietary glycemic load, carbohydrate intake, and risk of coronary heart disease in US women. *Am J Clin Nutr.* 2000 Jun;71(6):1455-61.

Obesity and Overweight for Professionals: Data and Statistics: U.S. Obesity Trends. <http://www.cdc.gov/obesity/data/trends.html#> 07 July 2011.

Siri-Tarino PW, Sun Q, Hu FB, Krauss RM. Meta-analysis of prospective cohort studies evaluating the association of saturated fat with cardiovascular disease. *Am J Clin Nutr.* 2010 Mar;91(3):535-46.

Siri-Tarino PW, Sun Q, Hu FB, Krauss RM. Saturated fat, carbohydrate, and cardiovascular disease. *Am J Clin Nutr.* 2010 Mar;91(3):502-9.

Vitamins and Minerals

Autier P, Gandini S., Vitamin D supplementation and total mortality: a meta-analysis of randomized controlled trials. *Arch Intern Med.* 2007;167(16):1730-1737.

Centers for Disease Control and Prevention (CDC). Prevalence of overweight and obesity among adults with diagnosed diabetes--United States, 1988-1994 and1999-2002. *MMWR Morb Mortal Wkly Rep.* 2004 Nov 19;53(45):1066-8.

Council for Responsible Nutrition, Washington, DC. CRN Comments on IOM FNB calcium and vitamin D DRIs (January 28, 2009). <www.crnusa.org/pdfs/CRN_Comments_IOM_FNB_cal cium+vitaminDDRIs.pdf> [Reviewed 07 July 2011].

Ginde AA, Liu MC, Camargo CA Jr., Demographic differences and trends of Vitamin D insufficiency in the US population, 1988-2004. *Arch Intern Med.* 2009;169:626-32.

Holick MF, Siris ES, Binkley N, et al., Prevalence of Vitamin D inadequacy among North American postmenopausal woman receiving osteoporosis therapy. J *Clin Endocrinolog Metab.* 2005;90:32-15-24.

Holick MF. Vitamin D deficiency. *N Engl J Med.* 2007 Jul 19;357(3):266-81.

Hollis BW. Circulating 25-hydroxyvitamin D levels indicative of vitamin D sufficiency: implications for establishing a new effective dietary intake recommendation for vitamin D. *J Nutr.* 2005 Feb;135(2):317-22.

Office of Dietary Supplements – National Institutes of Health. Dietary Supplement Fact Sheet: Vitamin D. (June 24, 2011). <http://ods.od.nih.gov/factsheets/VitaminD> [Reviewed 07 July 2011].

Vitamin D

Cooper Geoffrey M, Hausman Robert E, The cell: a molecular approach 3rd ed. 2004; Chapter 12: 494-508.

Haffer SM, D'Agostino R Jr,Mykkanen L,et al., Insulin sensitivity in subjects with Type 2 diabetes: relationship to cardiovascular risk factors: the insulin Resistance Atherosclerosis Study. *Diabetes Care.* 1999;22:562-568.

Saltiel AR, Olefsky JM, Thiazolidinediones in the treatment of insulin resistance and type II diabetes. *Diabetes.* 1996;45:1661-1669.

Harris MI, Klien R, Wellborn TA, Knuiman MW, Onset of NIDDM occurs at least 4-7 yr before clinical diagnoses. *Diabetes Care.* 1992;15:815-819.

Holick MF. Vitamin D deficiency. *New England Journal of Medicine.* 2007 Jul 19;357(3):266-81.

Hollis BW. Circulating 25-hydroxyvitamin D levels indicative of vitamin D sufficiency: implications for establishing a new effective dietary intake recommendation for vitamin D. *J Nutr.* 2005 Feb;135(2):317-22.

Kahn SE, Haffner SM, Heise MA, et al., Glycemic durability of rosiglitazone, metformin, or glyburide monotherapy. *N Engl J Med.* 2006; 355:2427-2443.

Lebovitz HE, Insulin secretagogues: old and new. *Diabetes Rev.* 1999;7:139-153.

UK Prospective Diabetes Study Group. UK Prospective Diabetes Study 16: overview of 6 years' therapy of type II diabetes: a progressive disease. *Diabetes.* 1995;44:1249-1258.

Medication and Vitamin D Deficiency

Ahmed W, Khan N, Glueck CJ,et al., Low serum 25 (OH) vitamin D level (<32 ng/ml) are associated with reversible myositis-myalgia in statin-treated patients. *Transl Res.* 2009 Jan; 153 (1): 11-6.

Kantola T, Kivisto¨ KT, Neuvonen PJ. Grapefruit juice greatly increases serum concentrations of lovastatin and lovastatin acid. *Clin Pharmacol Ther.* 1998;63:397-402.

Lee P, Greenfield JR, Campbell LV. Vitamin D insufficiency--a novel mechanism of statin-induced myalgia? *Clin Endocrinol* (Oxf). 2009 Jul;71(1):154-5.

Med Study Video Board Review of Internal Medicine 2006: 194-197.

The Cell

"Cell" 29 October 2008. HowStuffWorks.com. <http://www.howstuffworks.com/environmental/life/cel lular-microscopic/cell-info.htm> [Reviewed 07 July 2011].

Biello, D. (16 October 2006) Blind Relatives Prove Facial Expressions Are Inherited: Scientific American. <http://www.scientificamerican.com/article.cfm?id=blin d-relatives-prove-fac> [Reviewed 07 July 2011].

Freudenrich, Ph.D., Craig. How Your Brain Works. 06 June 2001. HowStuffWorks.com. <http://science.howstuffworks.com/environmental/life/ human-biology/brain.htm> [Reviewed 07 July 2011].

Hotchkiss, R. S., Strasser, A., McDunn, J. E., & Swanson, P. E. (2009). Cell Death. *New England Journal of Medicine.* 361(16), 1570–1583.

Optimal Nutrition

Barr SI, Murphy SP, Agurs-Collins TD, Poos MI, Planning diets for individuals using the dietary reference intakes. *Nutr Rev.* 2003 Oct;61(10):352-60.

Dietary reference intakes. Nutr Rev. 1997 Sep;55(9):319-26. <http://www.ncbi.nlm.nih.gov/pubmed/9329268> [Reviewed 07 July 2011].

U.S. Food and Drug Administration. How to Understand and Use the Nutrition Facts Label. 2004 Nov. fda.gov <http://www.fda.gov/Food/LabelingNutrition/Consume rInformation/ucm078889.htm> [Reviewed 07 July 2011].

Wilkinson DL, McCargar L, Is there an optimal macronutrient mix for weight loss and weight maintenance? *Best Pract Res Clin Gastroenterol.* 2004 Dec;18(6):1031-47.

Health and Vitality

Carroll, J. The Gallup Poll, "Stress More Common Among Younger Americans, Parents, Workers," Jan. 24, 2007.

Hannan MT, Tucker KL, Dawson-Hughes B, Cupples LA, Felson DT, Kiel DP. Effect of dietary protein on bone loss in elderly men and women: the Framingham Osteoporosis Study. *J Bone Miner Res.* 2000 Dec;15(12):2504-12.

Li Z, Treyzon L, Chen S, Yan E, Thames G, Carpenter CL. Protein-enriched meal replacements do not adversely affect liver, kidney or bone density: an outpatient randomized controlled trial. *Nutr J.* 2010 Dec 31;9:72.

Lustig, Robert H, 2009. Sugar: The Bitter Truth. [video] Available at: <http://www.youtube.com/watch?v=dBnniua6-oM> [Reviewed 07 July 2011].

Misra D, Berry SD, Broe KE, McLean RR, Cupples LA, Tucker KL, Kiel DP, Hannan MT. Does dietary protein reduce hip fracture risk in elders? The Framingham Osteoporosis Study. *Osteoporosis Int.* 2011 Jan;22(1):345-9.

Saad, Linda. Half of Americans Pressed for Time; a Third are Stressed Out. 03 May 2004. Gallup.com. <http://www.gallup.com/poll/11545/Half-Americans-

Pressed-Time-Third-Stressed.aspx> [Reviewed 07 July 2011].

What You Are Eating and Who Is Responsible

Heaney RP, Layman DK. Amount and type of protein influences bone health. *Am J Clin Nutr.* 2008 May;87(5):1567S-1570S.

Paddon-Jones D, Short KR, Campbell WW, Volpi E, Wolfe RR. Role of dietary protein in the sarcopenia of aging. *Am J Clin Nutr.* 2008 May;87(5):1562S-1566S.

Paddon-Jones D, Westman E, Mattes RD, Wolfe RR, Astrup A, Westerterp-Plantenga M. Protein, weight management, and satiety. *Am J Clin Nutr.* 2008 May;87(5):1558S-1561S.

Robert R Wolfe: Protein Summit: consensus areas and future research. *Am J Clin Nutr.* 2008 87: 1582S-1583S.

Victor L Fulgoni, III: Current protein intake in America: analysis of the National Health and Nutrition Examination Survey, 2003–2004. *Am J Clin Nutr.* 2008 87: 1554S-1557S.

The Straw That Broke the Camel's Back

Gladwell, Malcolm. The Tipping Point, 2000. [audio book]

Ziegler, T. R. (2009). Parenteral Nutrition in the Critically Ill Patient. *New England Journal of Medicine.* 361(11), 1088–1097.

Clinical Importance

Danesh J, Whincup P, Walker M, Lennon L, Thomson A, Appleby P, Gallimore JR, Pepys MB. Low grade inflammation and coronary heart disease: prospective study and updated meta-analyses. *BMJ.* 2000 Jul 22;321(7255):199-204.

Danesh J, Collins R, Appleby P, Peto R. Association of fibrinogen, C-reactive protein, albumin, or leukocyte count with coronary heart disease: meta-analyses of prospective studies. *JAMA.* 1998 May 13;279(18):1477-82.

Heron M, Hoyert DL, Murphy SL, Xu J, Kochanek KD, Tejada-Vera B. Deaths: final data for 2006. *Natl Vital Stat Rep.* 2009 Apr 17;57(14):1-134.

Cardiovascular Disease

Espenshade PJ, Hughes AL. Regulation of sterol synthesis in eukaryotes. *Annu Rev Genet.* 2007;41:401-27.

Hu FB, Willett WC. Optimal diets for prevention of coronary heart disease. *JAMA.* 2002 Nov 27;288(20):2569-78.

Hu FB. Are refined carbohydrates worse than saturated fat? *Am J Clin Nutr.* 2010 Jun;91(6):1541-2.

Iso H, Sato S, Kitamura A, Naito Y, Shimamoto T, Komachi Y. Fat and protein intakes and risk of intraparenchymal hemorrhage among middle-aged Japanese. *Am J Epidemiol.* 2003 Jan 1;157(1):32-9. Erratum in: *Am J Epidemiol.* 2004 Feb 1;159(3):318.

Leadbetter W. F., Burkland C. E. Hypertension in unilateral renal disease. *J Urol*, 1938, **38** : 611-626.

Liu S, Willett WC, Stampfer MJ, Hu FB, Franz M, Sampson L, Hennekens CH, Manson JE. A prospective study of dietary glycemic load, carbohydrate intake, and risk of coronary heart disease in US women. *Am J Clin Nutr.* 2000 Jun;71(6):1455-61.

Obesity and Diabetes

Centers for Disease Control and Prevention (2011). U.S. Obesity Trends. <www.cdc.gov/nccdphp/dnpa/obesity/trend/maps/> [Reviewed 07 July 2011].

Dhingra R, Sullivan L, Jacques PF, Wang TJ, Fox CS, Meigs JB, D'Agostino RB, Gaziano JM, Vasan RS. Soft drink consumption and risk of developing cardiometabolic risk factors and the metabolic syndrome in middle-aged adults in the community. *Circulation.* 2007 Jul 31;116(5):480-8.

Get America Fit Foundation (2011). Obesity Related Statistic in America. <www.getamericafit.org/statistics-obesity-in-america.html> [Reviewed 07 July 2011].

National Institutes of Health. (1998.). Clinical Guidelines the Identification, Evaluation, and Treatment of Overweight and Obesity in Adults. The Evidence Report. <http://www.nhlbi.nih.gov/guidelines/obesity/ob_gdlns.pd> [Reviewed 07 July 2011].

Prevalence of Overweight and Obesity Among Adults with Diagnosed Diabetes- United States, 1988-1994 and 1999-2002. *MMWR.* 2004; 53(45): 1066-1068.

U.S. Department of Health and Human Services. (2001). The Surgeon General's Call To Action To

Prevent and Decrease Overweight and Obesity 2001.
<http://www.surgeongeneral.gov/topics/obesity/calltoac
tion/CalltoAction.pd> [Reviewed 07 July 2011].

Memory and Dementia

Alzheimers Disease Research (2011). Plaques and
Tangles.
<www.ahaf.org/alzheimers/about/understanding/plaqu
es-and-tangles.html> [Reviewed 07 July 2011].

Thacker, N. A., Varma, A. R., Bathgate, D., Snowden,
J. S., Neary, D., & Jackson, A. (2002). Quantification of
the severity and distribution of cerebral atrophy
provides diagnostic information in dementing diseases.
<http://www.tina-vision.net/docs/memos/2000-007.pdf>
[Reviewed 07 July 2011].

Parkinson's Disease and Mood Disorders

Wurtman RJ, Hefti F, Melamed E. Precursor control of
neurotransmitter synthesis. *Pharmacol Rev.* 1980
Dec;32(4):315-35.

www.ingramcontent.com/pod-product-compliance
Lightning Source LLC
Chambersburg PA
CBHW070802270326
41927CB00010B/2255